a s y l u m

Daman Singh graduated in mathematics from St. Stephen's College, Delhi, in 1984. She went to the Institute of Rural Management, Anand, for further studies and worked in the field of development for twenty years. She is the author of two previous works of non-fiction: *The Last Frontier: People and Forests in Mizoram* (1996) and *Strictly Personal* (2014), a memoir of her parents Manmohan Singh and Gursharan Kaur. She has also written three novels: *Nine by Nine* (2008), *The Sacred Grove* (2010) and *Kitty's War* (2018). She lives in Delhi with her husband and dog.

DAMAN SINGH

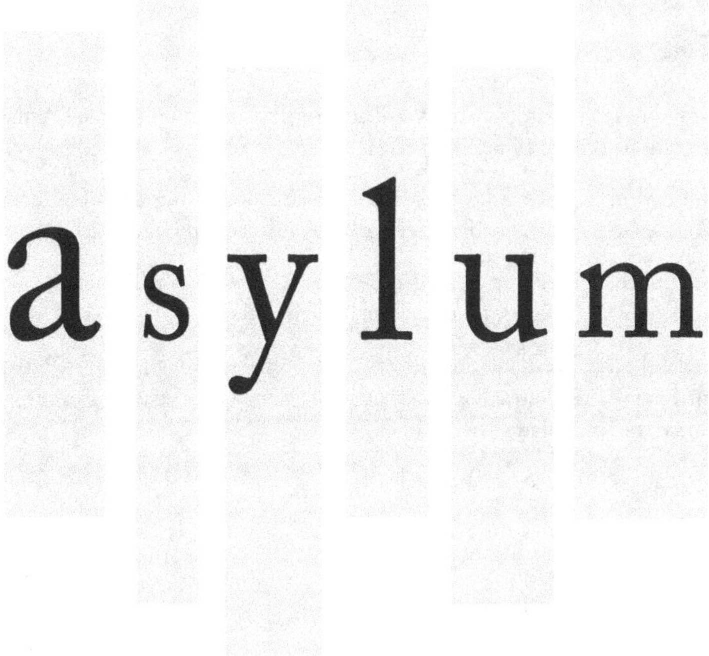

asylum

THE BATTLE FOR MENTAL HEALTHCARE IN INDIA

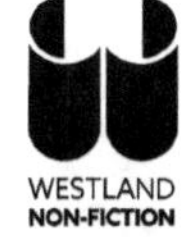

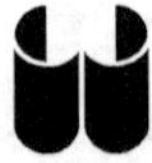

First published in hardback by Westland Non-Fiction, an imprint of Westland Publications Private Limited, in 2021

Published in paperback by Westland Non-Fiction, an imprint of Westland Books, a division of Nasadiya Technologies Private Limited, in 2023

No. 269/2B, First Floor, 'Irai Arul', Vimalraj Street, Nethaji Nagar, Alapakkam Main Road, Maduravoyal, Chennai 600095

Westland, the Westland logo, Westland Non-Fiction and the Westland Non-Fiction logo are the trademarks of Nasadiya Technologies Private Limited, or its affiliates

ISBN: 9789357764704

10 9 8 7 6 5 4 3 2

Typeset in Adobe Garamond Pro by SÜRYA, New Delhi
Printed at Saurabh Printers Pvt. Ltd.

Contents

Why Are We Here?

I have always been intrigued by the mysteries of the mind. These tend to crop up in much of what I read, and much of what I write. My first novel was about the unquiet mind. *Nine by Nine* came out in 2008. It was a quiet story of a young woman, Tara, who slowly loses her sanity. Reviews saw it as a coming-of-age story, a portrayal of life in a university hostel. Few, if any, noticed that Tara was mentally ill. This was a pity, but could not be helped. I moved on to write other books, on other themes.

In 2010, I happened to attend a seminar at the Nehru Memorial Museum & Library on the mental health aspects of communal conflict. It was the first of many organised by Dr Alok Sarin, a psychiatrist who was then a senior fellow there. A number of psychiatrists, psychologists, academics, and activists attended these seminars. As a mere writer, I was the least qualified of the lot. Pretty soon, I decided that I must learn all that I could about mental healthcare in India, past and present.

Ever since my last book appeared, various people have asked me what the next one would be about. There is an awkward silence after I tell them. Then they ask me why. 'Because,' I reply, 'nobody seems to have written the kind of book that I've been looking for.'

Asylum is that book.

When it comes to maladies of the mind, there is an enduring culture in the Indian subcontinent of turning to the occult, to faith, and to traditional methods of healing. In the 18th century, another option was added to this list – the lunatic asylum. The asylum was meant to protect society from the disturbing, disruptive, and possibly dangerous influence of the insane. It was a primitive form of captivity in cruel and barbaric conditions.

The first officially recognised – though privately run – asylum was established in Calcutta in the year 1788. Soon enough, public asylums came up across the breadth of British India. Foreign in both concept and design, the asylum became the approved place to confine the insane.

By the middle of the 19th century, medical science was thinking differently about insanity. The origin of this affliction was not yet clear. And its antidote was not yet known. But there was reason to believe that it could be corrected through humane and therapeutic treatment. As this view took root in the Western world, asylums began to be refashioned as institutions for the care of the mentally ill. While Britain was quick to attend to its own asylums, it took a while to turn to those in its largest colony.

This book is the story of asylum reform in India. It begins in the early 20th century, when the subcontinent was under colonial rule. And it continues through the course taken by an independent, sovereign nation. It is about the force of new ideas and the grip of old ones. About civil servants, doctors, journalists, lawyers, and judges who pushed for change. About the course of political events. And about the weight of international opinion.

Fragments of this story are scattered in archival records, official reports, court proceedings, academic journals, and news articles. But nowhere have these been pieced together in a way that speaks to ordinary citizens like me.

This is what *Asylum* tries to do.

A Note

The names of mental hospitals have changed over the years. They have also tended to get long and unwieldy. To simplify matters – for myself and for the reader – I refer to a hospital by its location. So what is today the Institute of Mental Health and Hospital, Agra, is simply 'Agra' in my book. I trust that the reader will figure out when I am referring to an institution, rather than a city. The city of Ranchi presents a peculiar problem. The European Lunatic Asylum, Ranchi, was set up in 1918. Then, the Indian Mental Hospital, Kanke, opened in 1925. Kanke is a suburb of Ranchi, and the two hospitals are practically neighbours. To get around this obstacle, I simply refer to the former as 'Ranchi' and the latter as 'Kanke'. Incidentally, 'Ranchi' is now the Central Institute for Psychiatry, Ranchi. And 'Kanke' has become the Ranchi Institute of Neuro-Psychiatry and Allied Sciences.

The names of a few cities have also changed with time. I have stuck to the first version that occurs in the book.

PART ONE

ONE

Asylum

In this country we are hardly ever called to see a patient in the initial stage … In the enormous majority we only see a patient when he is so insane, and has become so troublesome, that he is of necessity placed in an asylum to give security and freedom from annoyance to the sane population; even then, however, much can be done for the amelioration of many, and for the comfort and well-being of all.[1]

At the dawn of the 20th century, 8,365 men and 950 women were in asylums for the insane across British India. By Western standards, these numbers were absurdly small. There was no reason to believe that Indians were any saner than other people. So the asylums clearly contained only a fraction of all those who were mentally ill. Where were the rest?

They were, quite simply, at home, at large, or in jail.

A family was likely to overlook the early signs of mental illness in one of its own. If alarmed or anxious, it consulted tantrics and exorcists, pirs and fakirs, hakims and vaids. It tried

---

[1] G.F.W. Ewens, *Insanity in India: Its Symptoms and Diagnosis; with Reference to the Relation of Crime and Insanity* (Calcutta: Thacker, Spink & Co., 1908), 216.

tantra and mantra or potions and charms. It could also turn to beating, bleeding, and branding. Or to ropes and chains, bolts and locks. When all else failed, it might try its luck at an asylum – if indeed there was one within reach. But for that it would have to get a court order. It was easier to abandon its sick, perhaps at a place of worship. Or to look the other way when he – or she – just happened to wander off.

An unknown number of wanderers drifted about the countryside, fending for themselves. Some were seen as a public nuisance, others as a threat to public safety. The police could therefore round up beggars and vagrants. It could also round up those who seemed to be of unsound or deficient mind.

The legal system decided whether a person – produced by relatives or by the police – was eligible for admission to an asylum. This decision was taken by the police commissioner in Bombay, Calcutta and Madras city; and by a civil magistrate at other places. The authorities were assisted by a medical officer who was called in to examine the candidate. The doctor's job was to assess whether the person really was of unsound or deficient mind. And if so, whether he needed to be placed in state care. Someone who seemed to pose a danger to others, or to himself, was most likely to qualify. But other reasons might also play a part. The question called for a medical opinion and the answer was not always obvious. Especially if the doctor – like many doctors – had little experience to go by.

After that, it was up to the authorities. They could either order that the person be taken to an asylum. Or they could send him to jail for further observation. His spell in jail was not supposed to stretch more than a fortnight. But for a variety of reasons, it could last quite a while.

A harsher spell in jail was in store for those who were in for a crime. Some were convicts. Others had been acquitted on grounds of insanity. And then there were those who were yet to stand trial. All prisoners – sane and insane – had to submit to the discipline demanded in jail. But if a jail doctor certified that an inmate was insane, he was supposed to be transferred to an asylum instead. For a variety of reasons, this could take time.

In the year 1900, over a thousand persons were admitted to the asylums in British India. A few were brought in by family. One in four came over from jail. And the rest had been picked up from the streets.

~

The asylum was headed by an officer of the elite Indian Medical Service. As superintendent, this doctor was responsible for the diagnosis and treatment of those in his care.

Symptoms of mental illness varied a great deal in form as well as degree. For the purpose of diagnosis, a bunch of symptoms was labelled as a certain type of insanity. Three types of insanity were most reported – mania, melancholia, and dementia. Among patients admitted in the year 1900, around 61 per cent were described as manic, 19 per cent as melancholic, and 8 per cent as demented. What did these labels mean?

Outside the covers of medical textbooks, they meant different things to different doctors.

For Dr G.F.W. Ewens, the superintendent of the Lahore asylum, mania was the easiest to recognise. The patient was excited, restless, as easily moved to laughter as to tears. His thoughts flew and his speech was rapid, even incoherent. He was impulsive, defiant, and would not be reasoned with. High on energy, he slept very little. The acutely manic patient was oblivious to social niceties. He was noisy and abusive. He could tear off his clothes and go about naked. Being checked enraged him to the point of injuring himself, or those around him. Dr Ewens saw the melancholic patient as one who suffered from persistent misery. Solitary and still, he either remained silent or else he wept and wailed. He refused to occupy himself in any way, even to eat his meals. He was indifferent to his appearance and personal hygiene. He had no interest in life and might try to end it. The demented patient, in Dr Ewen's opinion, had lost his memory, intellect, and volition. Helpless as a child, he asked for nothing and generally did as he was told. He was very much like a mentally deficient person, except that his condition had come about late in life.

Through the 19th century, medical science was unable to figure out the cause of mental illness. It could not explain how human thought, feelings, and will were impaired. Nor had it come up with a cure for, say, mania, melancholia, or dementia. But this did not mean that mental illness could not be treated. It certainly could, and it was. But the remedies were not strictly medical. And the results could not be predicted.

In a case of acute mania, Dr Ewens believed that regular and ample feeding was essential – if necessary, by force. For a patient who did not take eggs and meat, he suggested plenty of milk, ghee, sago, tapioca, and rice. If also induced to perform some form of manual labour, certain patients became less violent and began to sleep better. Sedatives and hypnotics were useless in acute mania, but a heavy meal or warm bath might help. Dr Ewens found that the most effective way to deal with chronic cases of restless and violent behaviour was to leave the patient in the open – preferably in a grassy spot in the shade. If this did not work, the only option was to confine him in a separate room, with a large amount of straw to prevent him from injuring himself. At times he could also be administered a hypnotic such as sulphonal, chloral, potassium bromide, trional or veronal. Such drugs were of no value in a case of melancholia. A melancholic patient might, however, respond to large quantities of nourishing food, and to some form of exercise or occupation.

Dr Ewen's general prescription for most of his patients was liberal and regular nourishment, careful nursing, rest, exercise, and occupation. He also recommended that patients be treated with patience, politeness, and honesty. While his methods may have been in vogue at Lahore, they were not necessarily followed at other asylums. It was up to each superintendent to treat his patients in whatever way he thought best.

The asylums at Colaba, Lahore, and Madras were large, and running them was a full-time job. Elsewhere, an asylum was just one of the superintendent's many duties in the district. Though he visited it from time to time, someone else looked after day-to-day affairs. At Bhawanipur, Dullunda, Jubbulpore, Nagpur, and Tezpur, that someone was a junior doctor. But those who looked after the 15 remaining asylums did not hold a medical degree. Without a doctor at hand, the treatment and care of patients could become even more doubtful.

Nevertheless, every asylum reported that a number of patients recovered every year. Some were sent back to jail. And some were sent back home. But many would remain unclaimed for the rest of their life.

In the year 1900, around 11 per cent of the asylum population recovered. An equal number died.

~

Each asylum in British India was one of a kind. The one at Bhawanipur was simply a house to which barracks had been added later on. It could only accommodate 42 patients, and was reserved for Europeans and Eurasians. The Berhampore asylum was set up in abandoned military barracks. Dullunda was a circular building with a central courtyard surrounded by small rooms. The Madras asylum was very different. Dating back to 1871, its cottages and single-roomed blocks were set amidst spacious grounds. With a capacity of 689 patients, it was the largest of all asylums. Lahore was also different. Its construction was completed in the year 1900. And it was built on the lines of a prison.

The capacity of an asylum was decided by its floor space. Most asylums had a norm of 50 square feet per patient. Jubbulpore and Nagpur adopted a slightly higher norm of 54 square feet. Madras lowered the norm to 45 square feet in the section for Indians, and raised it to 60 square feet in the one for Europeans and Eurasians. At 72 square feet per patient, the most liberal norm was that of Lahore.

At times, the population of an asylum might exceed its capacity. In the year 1900, this is what happened in the men's quarters at Ahmedabad, Bhawanipur, Jubbulpore, Lahore, and Ratnagiri. Women's quarters at Ahmedabad, Dullunda, Jubbulpore, and Poona were also overcrowded; as were those of the Indian section at Colaba. Various other asylums were almost full for a part of the year.

Overcrowding was a serious problem. Cuttack had to transfer some of its patients to other asylums. And Agra and Benares had to stop accepting patients from jails. Due to the shortage of space at Poona, juveniles were kept with adult criminals, and recuperating patients stayed with those who were acutely ill. Civil inmates at Dharwar shared quarters with criminal inmates. And well-behaved patients were placed together with violent patients at Tezpur.

Most patients at Calicut and Madras were not considered violent. But a third of Vizagapatam's patients were reported to be so. Several such patients at Tezpur were confined in cells. Cells were also a common feature at Dharwar. At Dullunda, a patient managed to escape by picking the lock of his cell. Locks of the sort that were used in jails were installed after this incident. Three patients escaped through the bamboo fence at Tezpur. And one committed suicide by hanging himself.

Patients who were found fit to work were expected to make themselves useful at the asylum. A little less than half of Lahore's patients passed the test. At Agra, on the other hand, all the patients did. Usually, there was plenty of work to be done. This could include helping with cooking, grinding grain, plastering, and sweeping. Ten of the asylums had some amount of land suited to farming or gardening. There was a dairy farm at Bareilly, Dacca, Dullunda, Madras, and Patna. And an oil mill at Bareilly, Berhampore, and Jubbulpore. Some patients at Jubbulpore, Lahore, Madras, and Tezpur were engaged in weaving or tailoring. At Tezpur, women made most of the summer clothing for the patients. At Madras, European and Eurasian women were occupied with needle-work and knitting.

The monotony of asylum life might be broken by a variety of pastimes. Patients at Calicut played cards, chess, and other games. Several were allowed to keep pets. On one occasion, some of them were taken to watch an acrobatic show. On another occasion, they went boating and had a picnic. A sports gymkhana was organised at the asylum, where the public was admitted for a small fee. The *West Coast Spectator*, *Kerala Patrika*, and *Kerala Chandrika* were delivered to the asylum, free of charge. His Highness the Zamorin of Calicut and M.R.Ry. C.M. Rarichen Mooppen Avargal hosted 'treats' for the patients during the year.

Every Saturday afternoon, a Brahmin priest and a barber played music and sang at the Vizagapatam asylum. And troupes of actors, acrobats, and jugglers performed here through the year. The patients amused themselves at cards and chess, or with cymbals and tom-toms. A few of them were taken to the town to watch a play. The annual treat hosted by Sri Maharajah G.N. Gajapati Rao boasted a fireworks show, acrobatics, and gifts of fruit. The Rajah of Kurapam, Babu Nandi Lal Ghosani, and M.R.Ry. Motamarry Sanyasi Chetti Garu were the other benefactors that year.

The library in the Madras asylum was stocked with newspapers, periodicals, and books. Patients played football or croquet outdoors, and chess or draughts indoors. From time to time, jugglers, acrobats, bands, and performing bears were brought in to entertain them. Christmas was celebrated with a special treat. A Christmas tree was decorated and small presents were distributed.

A gramophone and records of English and Hindustani music were bought at Tezpur. Patients were provided with books, newspapers, musical instruments, and cards. The 'magic lantern' – or bioscope – was screened now and then. Sweetmeats and fruits were distributed on festivals. During Durga Puja, select patients were taken for the vashan ceremony at the river ghat. On another occasion, some were even escorted to the race course.

The mentally ill were vulnerable to a host of physical ailments. Many had been in a 'moribund' state when they arrived, and many would fall sick during their stay. Anaemia, debility, fevers, diarrhoea, dysentery, cholera, tuberculosis, and pneumonia were among the common ailments. Every asylum had an infirmary. Except for the one at Madras – which had trained nurses – all infirmaries were staffed by untrained attendants. As every infirmary did not have an isolation ward, infectious diseases were liable to spread. Sometimes such diseases travelled from the town to the asylum. In the year 1900, only 1 per cent of Ratnagiri's patients were in the infirmary on an average day. But the number was as high as 16 per cent at Madras. All said and done, it was a fairly healthy year at Cuttack, Dharwar, and Jubbalpore; and a fairly sickly one at Dacca, Dullunda, and Lucknow.

Some asylums took special precautions to keep their inmates healthy. For instance, 22 persons were being fed by tube at Madras and 9 were being fed by hand at Calicut. All patients were weighed once a month at Calicut, Dacca, Dullunda, Madras, Patna, Tezpur, and at Vizagapatam. At Vizagapatam, 59 per cent of the patients lost weight during the year. The figure was 47 per cent at Tezpur, 27 per cent at Madras, and 21 per cent at Calicut. Feeble patients were weighed more often and given extra food, tonics, and drugs. Better clothing was provided to convalescent and weak patients at Dacca, and warm clothes were issued well before the cold season set in at Lahore. Preventive doses of quinine were administered at both places. Tezpur dosed its patients with quinine, iron, and dilute sulphuric acid.

The Madras infirmary attended to 19 cases of injury that year. The injuries included a femur fracture after a fall from a verandah; bruising caused by an inmate banging his head against the iron bars of his cell; a scalp wound obtained while running; a cut received during an epileptic fit; a sore eye from being punched; and a bite on the back by a fellow inmate. Elsewhere, an elderly person sprained his knee while turning cartwheels. In a fit of excitement, one man fractured his collarbone, and another his ulna. And a woman was bitten by a snake as she tried to catch it.

Eleven per cent of the asylum population died in the year 1900. Jubbulpore had the lowest mortality rate of 2 per cent. The highest figure of 27 per cent was reported from Hyderabad in Sind province. Less than 5 per cent of the patients died at Agra,

Benares, Calicut, Cuttack, Dharwar, and Ratnagiri. On the other hand, over 20 per cent died at Ahmedabad and at Colaba that year.

In death as in life, no two asylums were alike.

~

Britain had an elaborate system to establish and administer its asylums. British India had nothing of the sort. And the flaws in its asylums were more than evident to those who cared to look within. Each asylum had its own peculiar history. Each was shaped by local circumstances. And each depended on how its superintendent chose to interpret his job. Outside of British India, much of the subcontinent was then under assorted Indian rulers. Little is known about the asylums in these territories. Many were simply jails by another name. But a few took their cue from the ones in the colony.

In January 1901, the *Indian Medical Gazette* carried a piece on the progress in the country during the past hundred years. Medical departments had been organised. Medical colleges and schools had come up. Hospitals and dispensaries had been opened. Diseases like small pox, typhus, cholera, and dysentery had 'lost their greatest terrors'. And research on malaria and typhoid was close to a breakthrough. The article said little about mental illness, except that its treatment was not as 'crude and rough' as it used to be. But it did make an important announcement:

We have on previous occasions referred to the changes which are about to take place in the management of the asylum in India[;] and with the new century we have every reason to expect that a new era is dawning for the insane in India.[2]

---

[2] Anon., 'Medical Progress in India during the Past Century', *Indian Medical Gazette*, vol. 36, no. 1 (January 1901): 22.

TWO

The New Era

It was a fortunate occurrence that before Lord Curzon left England to assume his duties as Viceroy[,] the requirements of Indian asylums were brought under his notice. He promised to look into the matter immediately on his arrival in India. Through a mutual friend, Dr McDowall was able to bring his presidential address under the notice of Lord Curzon. Whether owing to that fact or not, we now see the beginning of the reforms so urgently required.

… [W]e must heartily congratulate Dr McDowall on the achieved results of his labours. It is not often that a reformer commands instant attention.[3]

Having served in England's asylums for some thirty years, Dr T.W. McDowall was no stranger to insanity. Intrigued by a brief mention in a medical journal, he decided to find out more about its treatment in India. It was not possible for him to go there to see things for himself. So he relied on official documents and personal correspondence. What he learnt became the subject of his presidential address at the annual meeting of the Medico-

---

[3] Anon., 'Asylums in India', *The Journal of Mental Science*, vol. XLV, no. 191 (October 1899): 765, 767.

Psychological Association of Great Britain and Ireland in July 1897.

Though he called the colony 'a miracle' of successful governance in many respects, Dr McDowall said it was 'lamentably behind' in providing for the mentally ill. An asylum was under a medical officer who had neither specialised knowledge nor practical experience of the subject. He was burdened with exacting duties outside the asylum, and excessively occupied with routine tasks within. As he did not reside at the premises, the asylum was really run by his subordinates – an arrangement that was 'most vicious'. And after he had served but a brief tenure, a different medical officer would take his place. From this state of affairs, Dr McDowall expected nothing but 'evil and mismanagement'. According to his sources, asylums were both understaffed as well as underfunded. There were cases of 'very bare and miserable' accommodation, of overcrowding, of inadequate infirmaries, and of insanitary conditions. Dr McDowall believed that the system defeated the best intentions and killed the enthusiasm of the best officer.

Lord Curzon took over as Viceroy of India in January 1899. It appears that he actually kept his promise. Within a few months, Dr Robert Harvey, the Director-General of the Indian Medical Service, informed Dr McDowall that the government intended to reform the asylums in British India.

This was not a miracle. The government had been mulling over the matter for quite some time.

~

In August 1894, A.H.L. Fraser and Dr C.J.H. Warden submitted a confidential note to the government. A civil servant, Fraser was then divisional commissioner of Chhattisgarh. Warden was a professor of chemistry and also the chemical examiner at Calcutta. Both men had been members of the Indian Hemp Drugs Commission. Since hemp drugs were believed to cause insanity, the commission had visited every asylum, scrutinised records, and spoken to witnesses. Its 3,281-page report dealt with a wide range of subjects – including the cultivation of hemp, production and trade of drugs, and the social and moral effects of drug consumption. Of their own accord, Fraser and Warden chose to write a separate report on the asylums in British India. This was bound to create waves, and it did.

Declaring themselves to be 'very unfavourably impressed', Fraser and Warden wrote of the want of interest, of scientific treatment, and of systematic supervision. In general, superintendents had a 'superficial' understanding of mental disease and an 'imperfect' view of their duties. Failing to realise the importance of their work, they tended to relegate it to subordinate staff. This was quite evident in the 'worthless' statistics of insanity that they produced each year, and the 'laughable' case records of asylum patients.

The two commissioners went on to make a series of stinging charges. They had seen a patient suffering from acute mania, 'shouting and singing and raving in wild delirium' while grinding corn in the glaring light of an open shed. Another patient 'raving and furious' in acute mania, was chained to a tree in an open court. There was no attempt to segregate patients according to their mental condition. Convalescents were 'thrown together' with the acutely ill. And recovered patients were 'herded' with those in all stages of mental disease. This, according to the superintendent concerned, was not 'either dreadful in itself or possibly disastrous' for those of sane mind. Fraser and Warden also observed an autopsy being conducted in an open verandah. They pointed out that recent slaughterhouse regulations did not allow an animal to be killed in the presence of other livestock. Yet inmates of the asylum were allowed to watch as the dead body of a fellow patient was dissected. According to Fraser and Warden, such 'flagrant abuses' would not be allowed in an asylum managed on scientific lines.

Rather than pin the blame on individual officers, Fraser and Warden found fault with the system. A small asylum was most likely to be neglected as it was a minor part of a medical officer's many duties. This would not happen in a large asylum run by a full-time superintendent who had special training and experience. Subordinate medical staff were products of Indian medical schools that taught next to nothing about mental disease. This could be corrected if superintendents were to provide clinical instruction to medical students. Unlike other branches of medicine, insanity was not a subject of scientific enquiry in India. Qualified medical officers could well be encouraged to change that.

Fraser and Warden believed that it was incumbent on the government to improve the system of asylum administration. This, they argued, was as important for medical science and education as it was for those who were mentally ill.

It fell to the Surgeon-General of India to refute Fraser and Warden's charges. As a matter of fact, Dr W.R. Rice had put in several years as an asylum superintendent, and as an asylum inspector. In Europe, he pointed out, the asylum was an expensive and specially designed facility. It was run by a full-time officer with special training, who was 'sumptuously' paid and housed on the premises. Its medical assistants were well-trained, its warders and keepers were reliable, and its clerks were intelligent. Nothing of the sort was affordable in India.

It was, he argued, unfair to expect Indian asylums to be run on the same lines as 'at home'. More often than not, they occupied 'some old building' for which there was no other use. Superintendents had no special training to speak of, got little support from their staff, and were saddled with various other responsibilities. Yet, statistics of cures and mortality actually compared well with those in the United Kingdom. If the medical officers were indeed as 'careless and inefficient' as Fraser and Warden thought, surely this would not have been the case.

In short, Dr Rice denied that there was any serious defect in the system. That said, he agreed with all of the improvements that Fraser and Warden suggested.

The next step was to consult local governments. So, in March 1895, letters went out with copies of the note by Fraser and Warden, and a memorandum by Dr Rice. The memo proposed the merger of all existing asylums into five large facilities at central locations. It also outlined the design, construction, and staffing of a model central asylum.

Needless to say, the note by Fraser and Warden was not appreciated. Local governments denied that its allegations applied to any of their asylums. The government of Madras perused the note 'with much surprise'. Bombay took exception to the 'exaggeration' and 'sweeping statements' by the two authors. And as their 'practical acquaintance with asylum administration' could not be great, their conclusions from a 'rapid tour' were not 'of much value'. The North-Western Provinces and Oudh considered the 'strictures passed' to be 'undeservedly severe' and 'based on insufficient evidence'. But it did admit that considerable improvement was both desirable as well as possible.

The response to Dr Rice's memo was mixed. Bengal and Assam did not mind merging their asylums into a big one that was shared by the two provinces. Punjab was already thinking of combining its two asylums. But the North-Western Provinces and Oudh was only willing to abolish one of its four asylums.

Madras declared that the idea was simply not practical. The Central Provinces said it was too expensive. And Bombay insisted on retaining all of its asylums, though one or two might be relocated.

Local governments saw the point of a large asylum with a full-time superintendent. But their many misgivings were real. It would require a big plot of land at a suitable site. It would be costly to build, maintain, and run. It would be vulnerable to the spread of contagious and infectious disease. And it would take patients far away from their families and friends. Besides, a province might prefer to do things in its own way. Or it might be content to leave things as they were.

The question of training medical subordinates was less contentious. Madras province was keen to introduce a series of lectures by the superintendent of the Madras asylum at the local medical school. The North-Western Provinces and Oudh proposed that the Agra superintendent would lecture at the city's medical school. Bombay wished to train its subordinate staff at its chief asylum. Bengal did not see the point of adding a special subject to the heavy medical curriculum merely for the sake of few asylum employees. It later changed its mind.

As negotiations continued, the Government of India came up with a compromise. It decided that each of the five major provinces was to have a central asylum. These would be located at Agra, Lahore, Madras, Poona, and at an as yet unnamed place in Bengal. Each would be managed by a full-time superintendent. This officer would also provide instruction in the treatment of mental disease. But this did not mean that the small asylums would cease to exist. While some were to close down, the rest would carry on – under part-time superintendents – as before.

And so, even before Lord Curzon took over from Lord Elgin as Viceroy, a new central asylum was under construction at

Lahore. Alterations to the Agra asylum had been approved. And plans for three more central asylums were already under way. But their superintendents' salaries were not yet approved. This had to be done in London.

In January 1900, the new Viceroy's Council wrote to the Secretary of State for India in London. This letter outlined Fraser and Walden's note, Dr Rice's proposals, and the response from local governments. It listed the small asylums that were to close down. And it listed the large asylums that were to be created.

The success of the scheme would depend mainly on the 'ability and energy' of superintendents of the central asylums. It was thus necessary to appoint and retain 'thoroughly efficient' officers. The council suggested that such officers should be selected from the junior ranks of the Indian Medical Services. And that they be paid a gradually increasing salary that was enough to make them 'content and devote their whole career' to asylum work. While the financial details were still being worked out, the council proposed an average salary of about Rs 1,000 per month. If this was approved, the total cost of superintendence of all asylums – big and small – would go up by Rs 2,050 per month. Being 'strongly impressed with the need for reform', the council did not believe that this expense was excessive.

London cleared the council's proposal by the end of the year.

But for Fraser, Warden, and Dr McDowall, the new era for asylums in British India may not have come as and when it did.

～

The new era was quick to take off.

Luckily, the Madras asylum had been designed on what were then considered modern lines. Built in 1871, its several small pavilions or cottages were set in an open expanse of 66½ acres. It was already large enough for 689 patients. All it needed were repairs and a few additions to its buildings.

The old Lahore asylum had been branded for long as poorly located, badly ventilated, unsanitary, and generally beyond redemption. A new one was built at a better site with accommodation for 468 patients. Unfortunately, it resembled a high-security prison in design, with heavy double gates, sections divided by 15-feet high walls, and wards fitted with bars as well as cages. The new asylum opened in March 1900. With that, the old Lahore asylum and the Delhi asylum shut down.

Plans to upgrade the 39-year-old Agra asylum took shape between 1898 and 1900. These were influenced by the 'less repressive' style in vogue in the West. Renovation of the asylum was completed in 1905. Its capacity nearly trebled from 376 to 946 patients.

In 1874, the Berhampore asylum was established in military barracks that had since been abandoned. From a 'sanitary' point of view, it was now considered a good candidate for expansion. Construction work began in 1901 and ended in 1905. While the old asylum was meant for only 273 patients, the new one could take in 620. Thus, the Cuttack and Dullunda asylums closed, and their patients were transported to Berhampore. But at this point the government of Bengal 'reluctantly recognised' that the new facility was more suitable for a jail. After much thought, it decided to buy land in Ranchi, on account of the town's 'climate and healthiness'. The Berhampore asylum would have to carry on till a more modern one was built in Ranchi. Until then, improvements at Berhampore were more or less put on hold.

In 1913, a new asylum opened at Yeravda, near Poona. Spread over 30 acres, it could accommodate 386 patients. This allowed the old asylums at Colaba and Poona to close down.

Yeravda was better planned than the rest. It was, for instance, less like a prison and more suited to patient comfort. It even had electricity.

A little over a decade after the reforms began, five central asylums were up and running. In terms of architecture, none was close to ideal. But a beginning had been made. And a great deal had been learnt along the way. In the years to come, this would be put to good use at Ranchi.

From the very beginning, the Ranchi project was plagued by administrative and financial problems. The shortage of funds would worsen when World War I broke out. And the scarcity of building material during the war did not help either. The plan was therefore split into two.

In May 1918, a sixth asylum was added to the big five. It was meant exclusively for European and Eurasian patients from provinces in the north, east, and north-east. The Ranchi European Lunatic Asylum had been keenly awaited, as facilities for non-native patients were considered grossly inadequate. With a capacity of just 180 patients, it was the smallest of the central asylums. Public pressure pushed the government to open this asylum before it was fully equipped. As a result, it got bad press early on. Although conditions soon improved, the asylum would remain under the observation of English language newspapers.

Also located in Ranchi, the Indian Mental Hospital, Kanke, opened in September 1925 – seven years after its European counterpart down the road. The largest of all asylums in the country, it could take in as many as 1,378 patients. By the end of the year, 1,259 patients had been brought to Kanke in batches. With that, the Berhampore, Dacca, and Patna asylums were finally shut down.

The new era began with the creation of central asylums in British India. But it would take more than bricks and mortar to modernise the treatment of mental illness. For the most part, this task was left to the men who ran them. Who were these men?

The superintendent of a central asylum was to be an officer from the elite Indian Medical Service who had chosen to specialise in psychological medicine. He was to devote his entire career to asylum work. That is, he was to be an alienist.

In the early years, the alienists were few in number. Finding a suitable officer could take quite a while. And it could be difficult to find a suitable substitute when one of them went on long leave. As a result, a central asylum could – at times – be placed under a non-alienist. This problem was expected to sort itself out. It did.

Given its size, the Madras asylum had always been under a full-time superintendent. While Dr C.H.L. Palk had held charge since 1895, he went on long leave in mid-1901. A part-time officer took his place for the next two years. Dr Reginald Bryson served as superintendent from 1903 to 1908. He was then replaced by Dr P. Heffernan.

Dr G.F.W. Ewens was the first superintendent at the new central asylum at Lahore. He would serve till he suddenly died of angina pectoris in September 1914. Agra was under Dr A.W.R. Cochrane, whose term lasted from 1905 to 1911. After that, Dr A.W. Overbeck-Wright took over. Dr C.J. Robertson-Milne was in charge at Berhampore from 1906. On his untimely death from typhoid fever in 1911, Dr A.G.M. Peebles came in. And in 1913, Dr W.S.J. Shaw was appointed as superintendent at Yeravda.

By early 1914, the alienists had settled in at Agra, Berhampore, Lahore, Madras, and Yeravda. The situation would change dramatically when World War I broke out later that year.

As regards the administration of a Central Asylum, it should never be forgotten that the institution is primarily a hospital, and that it exists for the purpose of curing the insane or ameliorating their condition. At present the Superintendent is the only member of the staff who is required to be a specialist in mental diseases. In addition[,] therefore[,] to being obliged to carry out all the 'individual' treatment of the patients, and the laboratory work, he and he alone is responsible as Superintendent for the general management of the asylum.[4]

---

[4] W.S. Jagoe Shaw, 'Some Generalisations on the Scope, Construction and Administration of Central Asylums in India', *The Indian Medical Gazette*, vol. 49, no. 11 (November 1914): 426.

THREE

World War I

Over ten years have passed since the I.M.S. [Indian Medical Service] lost a member killed in action, the last being Captain F. Syme, killed at Gumburru, Somaliland, on 15th April 1903. It is curious that the first two I.M.S. officers killed in the present war should both be Indians, the first Indian members of the Service to fall in action, though Indians have served in the I.M.S. with credit and success for just fifty years.[5]

The first officers of the Indian Medical Service who were killed in action were Dr Pundit Piaraylal Atal and Dr Kunwar Indrajit Singh. Dr Atal had trained at St Bartholomew's Hospital in London. He joined the service in 1899. Dr Indrajit Singh had studied at Cambridge and at King's College, London. He entered the Indian Medical Service in 1911. The two men had been among the 54 Indian officers and 718 British officers in the service before World War I began.

The Indian Medical Service was a military organisation. Its recruits came through a competitive examination that was held

---

[5] Anon., 'Service and War Notes', *The Indian Medical Gazette*, vol. 50, no. 2 (February 1915): 75.

in London. Their main job was to serve the British Indian Army during war and during peace. Since their military duties were limited in peacetime, most were placed in top civil posts – until they were needed back in the army.

Just before the war, 443 of the 772 officers were in civil posts across the country. During the war, as many as 393 of them would be recalled for military duty. As the war raged at multiple fronts, it demanded more medical men. Much of the shortage was met by enlisting civilian doctors from the provincial medical services, and by taking in private practitioners. As many as 354 civilians were serving overseas on temporary commissions in the Indian Medical Service when the war came to an end.

With so many officers being plucked from top civil posts, medical services in the colony were bound to take a beating. This was tackled in all sorts of ways. Leave of absence was cancelled. Officers were assigned additional duties. Retired officers were rehired. Doctors from other services were inducted, and private practitioners were brought in. By the end of the war, 331 such outsiders were in civil posts vacated by officers of the Indian Medical Service. And a number of other posts had been relinquished to non-medical officers.

The depletion of medical personnel was not restricted to the officer class alone – it would also sweep down the rank and file. Some were requisitioned for military duty, others volunteered.

World War I left India's medical services in a state of disarray. It would take many years for the system to recover.

~

How did the central asylums fare during the war?

The Madras asylum had a long history of being led by an Indian Medical Service officer who was given no additional responsibilities. When Dr Heffernan left for military duty in April 1915, a retired officer from the service took his place. Dr C.H.L. Palk was not new to the asylum – he had earlier served as superintendent for several years. But after he left in early 1918, a series of doctors – part-time or full-time – from assorted services were in charge. Meanwhile, the asylum was hard-pressed for space, as batches of 'military insanes' began to arrive from the battlefront. This situation persisted well after the war came to an end.

In 1923, the Madras government decided to put an end to the practice of having a superintendent from the Indian Medical Service. Dr H.S. Hensman, an officer from the provincial medical service, was sent to train in psychological medicine in the United Kingdom. He returned to take charge as the alienist at the asylum.

For eight years after the death of Dr Ewens in September 1914, no officer of the Indian Medical Services – part-time or full-time – could be spared for the Lahore asylum. A junior doctor remained in charge during much of this time. Dr J.F. Fleming had to run the 800-bed asylum with virtually no medical staff. In early 1921, his health broke down under the strain and he passed away soon after. In 1922, an Indian Medical Service officer was back at Lahore. Dr C.J. Lodge Patch, an experienced alienist, took over as superintendent in November that year.

Lahore had been sorely stretched during the war. It saw a steady increase of patients, from 736 in 1914 to 876 in 1918. As many as 308 'military insanes' were admitted between 1917 and 1919. Temporary arrangements were made to deal with the overcrowding, while permanent measures were postponed for the future. The departure of both medical and non-medical staff for military duty left the asylum badly short of hands. And it was difficult to engage labour of any kind during the war years. In the past, a number of patients were kept busy making blankets, clothing, and mats. These activities had to be cut back due to the shortage of raw material, and the embargo on goods traffic.

At Agra, Dr Overbeck-Wright was recalled by the army in December 1914. His deputy took over for the next ten months, till he too left for military duty. A retired junior officer was then brought in for a few months. In February 1916, the asylum was added to the duties of the Indian Medical Service officer in charge of the district. Agra had to make do with a part-time superintendent till Dr Overbeck-Wright got back in June 1919.

The asylum had been overcrowded right through the war. Its population shot up from 625 patients in 1914 to 808 patients in 1918. A fair number of them were European and Anglo-Indian. These patients were supposed to be moved to the new asylum at Ranchi. But the Ranchi asylum was not ready till 1918. Agra saw its first 'military insanes' in 1916. The influx would continue till 1922. A major expansion of the asylum had been ruled out by the lack of funds. Patients had to be put up in a mill house and other old buildings. In the meantime, several patients seeking admission were either turned away, or directed elsewhere.

While Dr A.S.M. Peebles remained at Berhampore till December 1917, junior doctors at the asylum came and went right through the war. During the next six years, the superintendent's post changed hands a great many times. The asylum would be without an alienist till late 1923, when Dr J.E. Dhunjibhoy stepped in. Dr Dhunjibhoy had joined the Indian Medical Service in 1917 on a temporary commission, but had since been made permanent. He was the first Indian officer from the service to be appointed as an alienist.

The Berhampore asylum had been short of accommodation both before and during the war. It was supposed to be replaced by a new asylum at Ranchi. But the Ranchi project continued to be held up. And improvements at Berhampore continued to be put off. Overcrowding was an annual feature, and 'military insanes' added to the strain. Godowns and work sheds were converted into wards to deal with the growing number of patients. European and Anglo-Indian patients were finally taken to Ranchi in 1918. Indian patients, however, had to wait till 1925.

The Ranchi project had been delayed for many years. And the war delayed it further. Originally, the plan was for an asylum with one section for European and Anglo-Indian patients, and another section for Indian patients. Somewhere along the way, it was split into two separate projects.

The Ranchi European Lunatic Asylum opened in May 1918. This meant that European and Anglo-Indian patients at Agra and Berhampore would at last be shifted to a considerably better facility. The new asylum was a prestigious institution, and there were several keen applicants for the post of superintendent. The position finally went to Dr Peebles, who had put in a number of years at Berhampore. But two months into the job, Dr Peebles was recalled for military duty. The asylum was without an alienist till Dr O.A.R. Berkeley-Hill took over in October 1919.

All this while, the fate of the second asylum at Ranchi remained uncertain. The Indian Mental Hospital, Kanke, would only open in September 1925. That put an end to the old asylum in Berhampore.

Yeravda was the only central asylum to retain its alienist through the war. But Dr W.S.J. Shaw was no longer a full-time superintendent. He had various other demanding duties, including the hospital at the central prison.

When the asylum had opened in 1913, many essentials were yet to be added. Its facilities remained incomplete due to financial stringency during the war. Attracted by the better pay offered in the army, a number of warders and sweepers left the asylum. These employees proved hard to replace. Meanwhile, the number of patients went up from 339 in 1914 to 444 in 1918. 'Military insanes' had poured in, and overcrowding was persistent.

The war had dislocated the alienists, and disrupted the working of the central asylums. How did it affect the smaller ones?

The smaller asylums had always been run by part-time officers with no particular experience in psychological medicine. But the general instability in medical personnel, the financial curbs, and the interruption in supplies must surely have taken their toll. Perhaps this would partly explain why their average mortality went up by 2 per cent during the war.

∾

After the war, the Indian Medical Service was a much diminished organisation. By this time, the service was losing its appeal for British aspirants. Fewer candidates came forward to compete for vacancies. As a result, the entrance exam had not been held for quite a while.

Medical education in Britain had become more expensive. And there were plenty of well-paid jobs for medical men 'at home'. Besides, the political balance in the colony had shifted. There were reports of hostility towards foreign officers, and of demands that Indians take their place. Rumours hinted that the Indian Medical Service was about to be disbanded. Or that it was about to be flooded with Indian officers. In which case, British officers would be stripped of top civil posts – the main attraction in the service.

To some extent, the last of these rumours was true.

In 1919, the imperial government devolved some of its powers to the provinces. The provincial legislative councils were expanded, and the number of elected members was increased. Among other subjects, medical administration – including hospitals, dispensaries, asylums, and medical education – would now be under the provincial governments.

Within the boundaries of the Indian Lunacy Act, each province was now free to run its asylums as it wished. There was, however, one exception – the Ranchi European Lunatic Asylum, which was located in Bihar and Orissa province. This asylum was meant exclusively for white and semi-white patients from five different provinces. Their race set them apart from the 'native' population. This was sufficient reason to keep the asylum out of the hands of the provincial government. Under a special law passed in 1922, it was placed under a board of trustees whose members and functions were decided by the Government of India.

In the wrangle over provincial posts, the Indian Medical Service was bound to cede ground. But it managed to hold on to the superintendent's job at Ranchi and at Yeravda. Thus, Dr Berkeley-Hill would continue at Ranchi, and Dr Shaw would continue at Yeravda.

From 1923, the other four posts were thrown open to the provincial medical services. This could well have spelled the departure of three alienists – Dr Overbeck-Wright at Agra, Dr Lodge Patch at Lahore, and Dr Dhunjibhoy at Berhampore. But that did not happen. The provincial governments in question decided to keep all three officers where they were.

Dr Dhunjibhoy was then the least experienced of the three. Two years after he took over at Berhampore, the asylum was closed down. So were the ones at Dacca and Patna. In 1925, the patients of all three asylums were shifted to the brand new Indian Mental Hospital, Kanke. Dr Dhunjibhoy became the first superintendent of the largest asylum in the colony.

Madras province was the only one to make a clean break from the past. The provincial government decided to appoint one of its own doctors to head the asylum at Madras. In 1923, it sent Dr H.S. Hensman – a Tamilian of Ceylonese origin – to England, where he trained in psychological medicine for a year. He would take charge as superintendent of the asylum on his return.

~

By the early 1920s, each of the six central asylums had an alienist at the helm. All but one were being run by a provincial government. In the new scheme of things, would a provincial government pay adequate attention to the asylum? Would it fund the asylum fairly? Would it administer the asylum well? And would it respond to the needs of the local population? Indeed, it often did. But society as a whole was yet to voice a demand for better treatment of its mentally ill.

> General hospitals in India are up-to-date and wonderfully well constituted for the requirements and conditions of the country. The only reason that the asylums are not quite on the same footing is because there has been no popular demand for such institutions, largely due to the ancient and erroneous idea that mental disease is something occult and mysteriously ordained, and that treatment is quite useless.[6]

---

[6] W.S. Jagoe Shaw, 'Some Generalisations on the Scope, Construction and Administration of Central Asylums in India', *The Indian Medical Gazette*, vol. 49, no. 11 (November 1914): 424–425.

FOUR

The Alienists

In April last year[,] the Government of India issued a memo to the Local Governments[,] in which it was decreed that with the approval of the Local Government concerned[,] the name Mental Hospital could in future be substituted for Lunatic Asylum. I suppose that this change in nomenclature has meant very little to most people, but to those who had been doing all that lay in their power for years past to bring this change to pass, this memo of the Government of India brought immense delight, for it meant to them the inauguration of the first step towards the hospitalisation of the asylums in India and all that should follow from this, namely the beginning of an extended interest in psychiatry in all its branches.[7]

The first formal proposal to rename 'lunatic asylums' as 'mental hospitals' had come from Dr W.S.J. Shaw in 1916. Then the superintendent at Yeravda, Dr Shaw wrote to the Government of Bombay, pointing out that this was the trend in England as well as in America. The Government of Bombay supported

---

[7] Owen A.R. Berkeley-Hill, 'A Plea for the Inception of a Mental Hygiene Movement in India', *The Indian Medical Gazette*, vol. 58, no. 6 (June 1923): 242.

the idea and forwarded his letter to the Government of India. The Government of India wrote to all local governments and asked for their views. While some were against the change, a majority were in favour of it. The Government of India itself was not particularly enthused. It noted that the terms 'hospital' and 'asylum' were not synonymous. While a hospital provided medical treatment, an asylum was simply a place of refuge. And until the asylums in India were run by specialists – an event that was then considered a long way off – there was little to gain by calling them hospitals.

Still, the Government of India was ready to go ahead. As the change would require amending the law, it referred the matter to the legislative department. The legislative department did not consider it worthwhile to introduce legislation in wartime merely for the sake of a 'euphemism'. In 1917, the proposal was dropped.

Dr Shaw waited three years before bringing it up again. And this time he was backed by no less a personage than the Director General of the Indian Medical Service.

This time the change was not seen as a mere euphemism. In 1922, the Indian Lunacy Act was amended on the grounds that modern opinion was in favour of asylums being regarded as 'hospitals for the treatment of mental cases, and not as homes in which lunatics can be interned and restrained'. And, that it was desirable to emphasise the 'curative treatment which should be available in these institutions'.

After that, all local governments in British India could choose to rename their asylums. Every one of them did so. And so did the princely states of Baroda, Hyderabad, Mysore, and Travancore.

At home, Britain would outlaw the term 'lunatic asylum' eight years later.

∽

The alienists were a handful of doctors who had chosen to specialise in psychological medicine. These specialists were expected to turn lunatic asylums into mental hospitals.

All of the early alienists held British medical degrees. All of them were from the Indian Medical Service. And all of them were white.

As psychological medicine was part of the medical curriculum in Britain, the early alienists were familiar with the basics. Some had added to their knowledge and skills before they came to India. Dr Ewens, for instance, had spent some time studying the subject. Both Dr Overbeck-Wright and Dr Shaw had worked at mental hospitals in Britain. But not every alienist had this advantage. Those who were new to the field would therefore be sent 'home' for a few weeks of practical training. Various alienists were introduced to an Indian mental hospital by filling in for a superintendent who was on leave.

The second crop of alienists was different.

Since 1855, the Indian Medical Service had recruited its officers through an open competitive exam in London. As long as they held a British medical degree, Indian doctors were free to compete. Naturally, such candidates were limited to a privileged few. But more opportunities would open up when degrees from certain Indian universities were recognised – Bombay in 1892; Calcutta, Madras, and Punjab in 1893; Allahabad in 1914; and Lucknow in 1921.

Before World War I, there were 54 Indians in the Indian Medical Service. The number would rise during the war as civilian doctors were given temporary commissions. A few of these doctors would later be offered a permanent position in the service. One of them was Dr Dhunjibhoy. In 1923, he became the first Indian alienist in the colony. After serving as the superintendent at Berhampore for two years, he took charge of the Indian Mental Hospital, Kanke.

The second Indian alienist was Dr Hensman. Unlike Dr Dhunjibhoy, he was not from the Indian Medical Service. He was from the medical service of Madras province. Dr Hensman took over as superintendent of the Madras mental hospital in 1924.

Both Indian alienists held Indian medical degrees. As psychological medicine was not part of the medical curriculum in India, both officers were sent to train abroad.

Training in psychological medicine was not reserved for superintendents alone. In time, the provincial governments began to encourage their junior doctors to train in this field. When post-graduate diplomas in psychological medicine were introduced in the United Kingdom in the 1920s, a number of Indians would qualify. Dr Jyotirmay Roy, a deputy superintendent at Ranchi, earned his diploma in 1924. Five years later he would become the first full-time superintendent at Nagpur. Another diploma-holder, Dr Banarsi Das, took over at Agra when Dr Overbeck-Wright retired in 1934. A member of the Madras medical service, Dr Venkatasubba Rao had trained in America as well as in Britain in 1930. He had held a teaching position before coming in when Dr Hensman retired in 1936. As a deputy superintendent at Lahore, Dr Ram Singh Sharma had studied for the diploma in 1931. When Dr Lodge Patch retired in 1939, Dr Sharma would take his place as superintendent.

Indian alienists were not confined to British India alone. At least three princely states realised their worth. Then serving in the Maharaja's state of Mysore, Dr Frank Noronha had trained in London in 1922. He returned to work at the mental hospital in Bangalore, and became its superintendent in 1925. Armed with his diploma in psychological medicine, Dr A.S. Johnson took charge of the mental hospital in the Maharaja's state of Travancore in 1933. In the same year, Dr C.A. Sundar Raj was appointed to head the mental hospital in the Nizam's state of Hyderabad.

After World War I, all sorts of medical men were alienists. Some were white, others were brown. Some held a British medical degree, others an Indian one. Some were from the Indian Medical Service, others from the provincial medical services. Some were senior doctors, others were junior. And while some served in British India, others worked in the princely states.

All these alienists had one thing in common – they had trained abroad.

~

Psychological medicine was an emerging field, and advances were being reported from eminent institutions across Europe and America. For the alienist in India, white or brown, a study tour to such places was both instructive as well as inspiring.

In 1931, Dr Banarsi Das travelled to France, Germany, Holland, and the United Kingdom. His trip was supported by the United Provinces government. And it was planned with the help of Dr A.E. Evans, a member of the Board of Control for Lunacy and Mental Deficiency at London.

In 'A Psychiatric Tour of Europe', an article for *The Indian Medical Gazette*, Dr Das spoke of mental hospitals with modern buildings, extensive grounds, and up-to-date equipment. He also described clinics for the early treatment of outpatients, and laboratories engaged in biochemical research. Some of the new treatments he got to observe were electric therapy and hydrotherapy in Berlin, malaria therapy in Vienna, and 'active therapy' at the provincial hospital near Santpoort in Holland.

The 'non-restraint' system in Britain and in Holland seemed to have made quite an impression on Dr Das. Holland, he noted, had made great progress in treating mental illness, despite its small size. Calling it a 'charming country of dykes and windmills', he confessed that he had never seen 'so many bicycles *en masse* anywhere'. He was particularly taken with the 'thoroughness and attention to detail' at German clinics. At the Sainte-Anne hospital in Paris, he was struck by the life-sized statues adorning the wards and passages, and the murals painted by patients. 'Apparently,' he remarked, 'the French temperament finds special solace in art, even when reason is clouded.'

'A Psychiatric Tour of Europe' took care to mention some of the personalities whom Dr Das had met. They included the superintendent of the Oxford mental hospital, a man of 'unbounded enthusiasm'. Then there was the director of Den Dolder, 'a thorough-going Freudian'. At his institute for brain research in Vienna, Dr Constantin von Economo – who had discovered sleeping sickness – showed Dr Das casts of brains made with 'some secret composition' imported from Switzerland. But Dr Das reserved the greatest appreciation for Prof. Wilhelm Weygant, the director of the state mental hospital at Hamburg, and head psychiatrist at the university clinic.

Dr Das had turned up at Prof. Weygant's 'famous' clinic 'without any credentials'. In his broken German, he then asked the hall porter if an English-speaking doctor could show him around. To his surprise, the director offered to do so himself. It so happened that Prof. Weygant had actually studied Sanskrit, and was also familiar with 'Indian affairs'. He spent a great deal of time conducting Dr Das through his 'wonderful museum of brains and skulls, of not only all living and extinct races of man, but also of every animal from the smallest to the biggest'. After that, one of his assistants took Dr Das around the hospital and laboratories. This was not all. Prof. Weygant gave him letters of introduction to directors of the clinics at Berlin, Vienna, Munich, and Paris.

Like Dr Das, Dr Dhunjibhoy had toured mental hospitals and clinics in Europe as a newcomer. By the time he set off on his second trip in 1929, he was already an experienced alienist. He spent all of six months of study in London, before visiting some of the 'most modern' facilities in England, Belgium, France, Germany, and Vienna. The trip was not just about learning, he also had much to share. He was invited to read a paper at a meeting of the Royal Psychological Association of Great Britain and Ireland, held at Cheshire in England. A similar request came from the Hospital Charité in Berlin. In 1930, Dr Dhunjibhoy also travelled some 3,000 miles across Canada and America. 'Thoroughly impressed' with what he saw in America, he believed that no other country had made 'such rapid progress in mental science'.

Dr Dhunjibhoy made another trip to America in May 1930. This time the Government of India sent him to Washington, DC as its delegate for the first international congress on mental hygiene. The conference was attended by 3,500 delegates from 53 countries. This 'epochal' event enabled Dr Dhunjibhoy to meet 'the world's celebrities in the field of psychological medicine'. He used the occasion to visit various institutions that he had missed on his previous trip.

On a longish trip that began in 1935, Dr Dhunjibhoy looked at methods of occupational therapy in England, Holland, and Germany. In Budapest, Dr Ladislaus von Meduna – a 'friend and colleague' – invited him to see his newly created convulsion therapy. And in Vienna, Professor Ernest Lowenstein explained his work on the link between tuberculosis and schizophrenia. Dr Dhunjibhoy would use these therapies at Kanke.

The value of study tours was best expressed by Dr Dhunjibhoy. He declared that there was no better way to greater knowledge and experience than meeting with outstanding experts in Europe and America.

~

While the alienists kept up with foreign books and journals, they also indulged in a fair amount of writing themselves. This would build a body of medical literature for students and practitioners in the country. Dr Ewens was the first to write a book for doctors working in India. *Insanity in India: Its Symptoms and Diagnosis, with Reference to the Relation of Crime and Insanity* came out in 1908. An authoritative volume replete with illustrative cases, it drew upon his early experience at Lahore. This book was followed by two authored by Dr Overbeck-Wright. *Mental Derangements in India: Their Symptoms and Treatment* appeared in 1912, and *Lunacy in India* in 1921. *A Clinical Handbook of Mental Diseases* by Dr Shaw was published in 1925. Dr Lodge Patch wrote *A Manual of Mental Diseases: A Textbook for Students and Practitioners in India* in 1934. He also wrote *A Critical Review of the Punjab Mental Hospitals from 1840-1930*. This insightful monograph was the only institutional account of its kind. A seventh publication followed in 1935. *Modern Methods in Psychiatry* was written by Dr J.N.J. Pacheco. Unlike the authors who came before him, Dr Pacheco was not from the Indian Medical Service. Nor was he British. He was an Anglo-Indian officer who served as a deputy superintendent at Ranchi for several years.

Foreign journals such as *The Lancet*, *The British Medical Journal*, and the *Journal of Mental Science* would occasionally offer articles by alienists in India. Back at home, *The Indian Medical*

Gazette was widely read by the medical fraternity. It carried extracts from the annual reports of India's mental hospitals, and reprinted pertinent pieces from foreign journals. In October 1914, it brought out a 'special insanity number'. In view of the enthusiastic response that came in, its coverage spilled over to the November issue as well.

Among the alienists, Dr Berkeley-Hill was easily the most prolific contributor to the *Gazette*. An avid reader, he also reviewed books for the monthly. Dr Berkeley-Hill's opinions about books and their respective authors were peppered with his characteristic wit, humour, and sarcasm. Other alienists who contributed articles in plenty included Dr Ewens, Dr Overbeck-Wright, Dr Heffernan, Dr Dhunjibhoy, and Dr Naronha.

The pages of *The Indian Medical Gazette* allowed a lively exchange of views between alienists, and between alienists and non-alienists. The latest theories of psychology, for instance, and methods like psychoanalysis, evoked strong opinions from readers. Dr Overbeck-Wright and Dr Berkeley-Hill would take opposing sides in this particularly sharp debate.

~

In due course, Ranchi and Kanke took to training their doctors in-house. Their next step was to train doctors from various other institutions. This feat was accomplished by Dr Berkeley-Hill at Ranchi, and by Dr Dhunjibhoy at Kanke.

The University of London offered a postgraduate diploma in psychological medicine, which required a period of practical training. In 1922, it recognised Ranchi as a centre for such training. This would encourage candidates from India to qualify for the diploma. The university gave the same recognition to Kanke in 1936. So did the University of Edinburgh.

Through the 1930s, an assortment of doctors headed to the European Mental Hospital at Ranchi for training. They included military officers and civilians, government employees and private practitioners. And they came from British India, from the Indian princely states, and from neighbouring countries too.

Before taking charge as the first full-time superintendent at Tezpur in 1933, Dr S.N. Chowdhury trained for six months at Ranchi. Two members of the Nepal medical service took a five-month course in 1934. Captain Ahmad, the police surgeon of Calcutta, attended a one-month course the same year. In 1935, Dr Hari Das Misra of the Bhopal State Medical Service joined in for staff lectures on the central nervous system, physiology, and psychology. In 1942, a three-month course was organised for three doctors. One was Dr S.K. Chakravarty of the Assam medical service. The second was Dr D.M. Batliwala, superintendent at the mental hospital in the princely state of Baroda. And the third was Dr J. Biggar, a private practitioner in Calcutta. With the outbreak of World War II, the hospital was requested to extend its training services to the military. Two such courses took place in 1943–44. They were attended by six military officers, and a civilian medical officer from the United Provinces. The following year, medical officers from a number of mental hospitals were instructed in shock therapy. And during 1945–46, the deputy superintendent at Yeravda, Dr I.K. Mujavar, would also take instruction from Ranchi.

The Indian Mental Hospital, Kanke, was the youngest – and by far the largest – of all mental hospitals in the country. Within a decade of its existence, it began to train doctors deputed by the government of Bengal. Dr Muhammad Husain and Dr Rajendra Chandra Das came over in 1935, and would remain for a period of two years. They were followed by Dr Amulya Mohan Sen and

Dr Atul Chandra Bhattacharjee in 1937, and by Dr S. Goswami in 1939.

While doctors had to wait till the 1930s to train at Ranchi and Kanke, a tiny beginning in medical education had been made much earlier. When central asylums first came up, one of the duties of each superintendent was to give a course of lectures and clinical demonstrations to students of provincial medical colleges and schools. As the alienists were few in number, this was only possible on a small scale. But by 1932, they would be joined in this task by superintendents at Ahmedabad, Bangalore, Bhawanipur, Hyderabad in Sind, Thane, and Vizagapatam. Taken together, these doctors were instructing students of 11 of the 13 medical colleges, and 12 of the 26 medical schools in British India.

～

In 1933, alienists were in charge at eight of the 17 mental hospitals in British India. This was by no means a big number. But since these hospitals were relatively large, they accounted for 74 per cent of all patients.

The alienists were trained to manage a mental hospital on modern lines. But it would not be easy for these specialists to put their training into practice. They had to scrounge around for funds. Their medical subordinates were by and large untrained. They were generally short of skilled and unskilled staff. Their concerns were rarely shared by the medical fraternity. And they had to contend with archaic notions about mental illness that pervaded the bureaucracy, the judiciary, the police, and the public.

While some efforts of the alienists would pay off, others

would peter out. Their successes and their failures drew attention to the flaws in the system. And they demonstrated what a lone alienist could – and could not – achieve.

> If ... [his superior] be inclined to take the proper view of his position the Suptdt. finds himself given consideration as expert and adviser in all things pertaining to asylums. His proposals & schemes for modernising his own asylum are given proper consideration & he is consulted on schemes for the district asylums ... This I submit is the position intended for him by the Govt. of India, but it is not always attained.
>
> After five years of such a regime a change occurs & a new Inspector General of Civil Hospls. is appointed. He is wedded to the old views regarding asylums & utterly fails to grasp the innovations ... and the changes ... necessary in asylums & the mode of treatment of the insane. In such circumstances, at present, all progress is not only suspended but the little already made is ruthlessly eradicated. Suptdts. may, & do, protest but of what avail is protest in such case. They can but tend their patients as best they can under wholly unsuitable conditions & hope that the next change may be a better one for their asylums & and the poor sufferers for whom they are responsible.[8]

---

[8] A. Overbeck-Wright, Note on the alienist department in India, dated 5 January 1919, DGIMS/ Medical section/ IMD, File no. 502, April 1918, National Archives of India.

FIVE

Bending the Rules

In other words, Psychiatry in India is now in the same position as it was in Europe fifty years ago – that is to say – as far as the bulk of the Indian population is concerned. Without in any way minimising the peculiar difficulties which arise, and which are due to the different standards of conduct, ethics, and religion … there is little doubt that Indian alienists start with a tremendous advantage over their European brethren of fifty years ago. There are not the same fallacious dogmas to forget, the same vicious practices to eschew; while there is much indeed to learn, there is at least little to unlearn.[9]

India's alienists were well aware of the principles of modern mental hospitals. But the hospitals were bound by rules that were anything but modern. Standard rules dictated how a hospital had to be administered. And unwritten rules based on convention – or convenience – indicated how it ought to run.

The alienists would need both grit and gumption to do things differently.

~

---

[9] P. Heffernan, 'The Voluntary Boarder', *The Indian Medical Gazette* (November 1912): 434.

Lahore had been without an alienist for eight years when Dr C.J. Lodge Patch arrived in 1922. Having worked at an 'up-to-date' mental hospital in Scotland for three years, he was eminently qualified for the position. This, however, did not prepare him for his stint as superintendent at Lahore. The very sight of the hospital was like 'a blow between the eyes'. It appeared to be a 'grim and grisly refuge for the insane'. And its patients were truly 'under a reign of terror'. Dr Lodge Patch was appalled at the rampant use of 'instruments of torture' such as handcuffs and fetters. He was also appalled by the long hours of isolation that many patients were forced to endure.

Early reports from Lahore had often stressed that several of its patients were violent. One went so far as to say that that every patient, no matter how quiet, 'must be looked upon as being, at some time, potentially dangerous'. Added to that, many had 'filthy habits', were 'constantly noisy', tended to 'annoy or bully' other patients, or were 'addicted to sodomy'. Such inmates were seen as a major problem in the shared barracks at night. The solution was to build a massive number of single cells and cubicles where each would sleep alone. In 1911, there were as many as 200 such enclosures. By the time Dr Lodge Patch took over, these enclosures were also in use during much of the day. Occupants were kept under lock and key while attendants took a lengthy mid-day break. The 'dangerous' ones among them remained in solitary confinement, day and night. All these patients had no option but to urinate and defecate in an open drain that ran through their cells.

While a superintendent was generally advised to adopt the 'non-restraint system' that was favoured in Britain, this was not spelled out in government rules. In theory, the decision to restrain or isolate a patient was supposed to be made on medical grounds alone. In practice, other reasons might come into play.

What kind of patient should be restrained or isolated? When were these measures justified, and for how long? How were difficult patients to be handled? None of these questions had an explicit answer. It was up to the alienist to figure things out. And to find a way to make them work.

One of the first things that Dr Lodge Patch did was to round up about a hundred kilograms of handcuffs and fetters and send them to the jail next door. He then put an end to the routine isolation of patients. Attendants were no longer allowed to take extended breaks during the day. Under no circumstances could they lock up any patient in a cell between 6 a.m. and 6 p.m. without a direct order from a medical officer. They were to treat all patients with 'the utmost kindness, consideration, and courtesy'. And anyone who flouted these instructions a second time was liable to be dismissed.

These changes called for better supervision, and for a better calibre of attendants. After the war it had become possible to recruit a class of demobilised sepoys of 'good character'. These men were used to military discipline, and were intelligent enough to grasp the nature of their new duties. Dr Lodge Patch also introduced a fifteen-minute 'infantry drill' twice a day. The new recruits took to this at once. Thus outshone, the clout of the old guard began to wane. In the space of about a year, the 'senior undesirables' had been weeded out. What then remained was an 'exceedingly smart and well disciplined' staff that proved to be 'most loyal, trustworthy and reliable'.

Dr Lodge Patch reported that when patients were treated humanely, they became far less aggressive and much easier to manage. This principle was, however, not followed everywhere. Decades later, mechanical restraint and isolation would still persist in several mental hospitals across the country.

∼

Prison reforms in 19th century Britain took the view that mentally ill inmates ought to be kept in facilities that provided suitable treatment. Towards the end of the century, this sentiment was echoed in British India. As a result, a number of mentally ill persons began to be transferred from jails to mental hospitals – or asylums, as they were then known.

In official parlance, these persons were initially called 'criminal lunatics', and later labelled as 'criminal insanes'. However, not all of them had been convicted of a crime. In Bengal, for instance, 65 per cent of the 1,043 'criminal insanes' transferred between 1890 and 1900 were yet to be tried in a court of law. Around 19 per cent had been acquitted by reason of insanity. Only 16 per cent were convicted felons.

A mentally ill convict would remain at the hospital until he recovered. But even after recovering, a person acquitted by reason of insanity had to put in at least three years of probation. The case of an undertrial was very different. Whether or not he had recovered, he was transferred back to jail once he was fit to appear in court. He was then kept in jail as long as his trial was on. If found guilty, and still mentally ill, he was sent back to the hospital, this time as a convict. If acquitted on grounds of insanity, he still returned to the hospital – for treatment and probation, or for probation alone.

Life in the hospital was nowhere near as harsh as it was in jail. But unlike other patients, 'criminal insanes' were subject to rules that were similar to those for inmates of a jail. These rules ordered strict confinement, and complete segregation from 'non-criminals'. In practical terms, they called for a jail within the hospital – an idea that found many willing takers. But Dr Ewens was not one of them.

As Lahore's first alienist, Dr Ewens had observed that most 'criminal insanes' behaved in a manner that was considered either improper, indecent, immoral, or criminal in normal people. If they did commit a violent act, it was usually sudden, impulsive, and bizarre. Their provocation or motive, if any, was childish and irrational. And acts of brutality against family members were not uncommon. In his opinion, sane criminals did not behave this way.

Dr Ewens therefore viewed the 'criminal insane' as a victim of insanity, rather than the perpetrator of a crime. He found that even those who had committed 'some horrible murder' while insane, proved to be 'quiet' and 'respectable' once they improved. So, except for the fact that they were in a separate compound, they were treated like all other patients. And 'everything reasonable' was done to make them 'comfortable and contented'. During 'sane intervals' and probation, many proved to be 'most trustworthy, reliable assistants and workers'. They did most of the cooking, operated the machines, and tended to the sick – far better, in fact, than the hospital attendants.

Later on, similar views were voiced by other superintendents – alienist and non-alienist alike. A number of them were particularly concerned about the 'harmless criminal insane' who had been charged with a trivial offence. Trivial offences could include petty theft, travelling without a railway ticket, indecent exposure, wandering into someone's house or compound, even 'kicking someone on the shin'. An earnest superintendent would try to convince local magistrates to drop such charges. If that was done, the person could remain as a civil patient, or might even be discharged. Some superintendents also urged the local government to tell magistrates not to charge mentally ill persons brought before them with trivial offences, but to send them in as civil patients instead.

The confinement of a 'criminal insane' was only partly in the hands of the superintendent. It was defined by the rules of the criminal justice system, and shaped by the manner in which these rules were applied. Till close to the end of the 20th century, neither was sought to be corrected.

~

The Indian Lunatic Asylum Act of 1858 was a very short law that basically dictated how a civilian was to get in and out of a mental hospital. In 1912, it was replaced with the Indian Lunacy Act. The new law was simply a detailed version of the old one, with certain added sections from other laws that dealt with 'criminal insanes' and 'military insanes'. Only one of its features was entirely original – the treatment of 'voluntary boarders'.

The idea of 'voluntary boarders' was to encourage people to come forward for treatment at an early stage of illness. This was already happening at various places in America, Australia, France, Germany, Italy, and the United Kingdom. But for India, it was nothing short of revolutionary.

Under the Indian Lunacy Act, a person could actually ask to be admitted for treatment of his own accord. And at any stage of his treatment, he could decide to end his stay. Unlike all other patients, a 'voluntary boarder' did not have to go through the rigmarole of a court order. Nor was he subject to the will of relatives, magistrates, or hospital authorities.

Berhampore saw just one voluntary patient in 1914. Another followed in 1917. And then four more in 1918. Dr Peebles was disappointed. Many 'well-to-do people' had asked him about the procedure for admission. He confessed that he did not know why so few of them came in.

The reasons were not hard to fathom. A voluntary patient would naturally expect facilities of a certain quality. Living conditions in most hospitals were basic, if not downright primitive. And the squeeze on budgets would tend to keep them that way. Besides, many hospitals were hard-pressed for space. Kanke, for instance, was often forced to turn away a large number of certified cases. Taking in voluntary patients was simply out of the question.

Madras was the first mental hospital to make headway. Within months of the new law being passed, five persons had asked to be admitted. The number was small, but as Dr Heffernan pointed out, 'Rome was not built in a day'. He believed that the scheme had come at a most 'opportune time' and it behoved all concerned to 'try and make it a success'. Wisely, he anticipated difficulties in providing suitable accommodation and medical care. But he thought that these would gradually 'yield to time and perseverance'.

By late 1914, the hospital had treated 34 voluntary patients from different walks of life. Among them were seven men of the 'liberal arts and professions', four of the 'landed gentry', and two merchants. Of the four European and Anglo-Indian women, two were teachers, and one was described as a 'mission agent'.

The effort to encourage voluntary patients continued under Dr Hensman. And sure enough, the numbers did pick up. Between 1912 and 1932, as many as 153 men and 27 women had come forward for admission. Two-thirds of them were Indian.

When the European mental hospital opened at Ranchi, the response was even better. This was not surprising. Ranchi had been built keeping in mind the needs of a 'better class' of patients. In fact, the eminent psychiatrist Dr Edward Mapother pointed out that it was like the less-expensive private hospitals in England. Such high standards, he felt, were really not necessary for white or semi-white people who lived in India. Ranchi treated 340 voluntary patients between 1921 and 1936 – an average of 21 persons a year.

After struggling for some decades, Yeravda was also able to offer special facilities for voluntary boarders. Elsewhere, only stray patients would show up.

~

Dr Berkeley-Hill took over at Ranchi in October 1919. A few months later, he was on the verge of being dismissed from the Indian Medical Service.

Soon after his arrival, Dr Berkeley-Hill had proposed a number of improvements at the hospital. But the Bihar and Orissa government continued to sit on his requests. Finally, he took the drastic step of going to the press. *The Statesman*, a prominent daily published in Calcutta, carried a biting piece on the condition of the hospital. This did not go down well in official circles. To keep his job, Dr Berkeley-Hill was forced to apologise for his 'improper conduct'.

But the story did not disappear. It was picked up by the Calcutta branch of the European Association of India. In June 1920, this influential group sent a two-member team to investigate. A flurry of activity soon followed. The association sent its report to the provincial government. J.V. Jameson, a member of the Bihar and Orissa legislative council, raised the subject in the house. The president of the association came over to see things for himself and called for an official enquiry. *The Englishman* printed a lengthy letter written by Jameson. Titled 'God's Convicts', it summed up for readers the 'unsatisfactory' state of affairs. And in October 1920, the association took up the matter with the Government of India. All this publicity would make it easier for Dr Berkeley-Hill to have his way.

Ranchi's clientele was a class apart. On the British social ladder, white and semi-white persons settled in India were – at best –

middle-class. But in colonial society they ranked as elites. In 1939, Ranchi would open its doors to another kind of elite. Under 'certain conditions' a few Indians 'of European habits' could also be admitted.

The hospital was clearly a cut above the rest. It was better designed, better built, and better equipped. It also enjoyed the kind of freedom that others did not have. From 1922, the hospital was no longer managed by the provincial government. Instead, it was governed by a board of trustees, in line with rules that were set by the Government of India.

Given its profile, Ranchi was the best place for an alienist who wanted to make a difference. Dr Berkeley-Hill, who served here till he retired in 1934, was a forceful personality, and a man of many ideas. During his tenure, the practice of restraint and seclusion of patients was abolished. Virtually all patients could get permission to leave the hospital – unescorted – during the day. Dr Berkeley-Hill did not believe in keeping men and women patients perpetually apart. So a variety of common recreational activities were organised for all patients. Before a patient was formally discharged, he could be sent home on 'leave of absence' for two months. This would test if his family was ready for him, and if he was ready for the outside world. When a more vulnerable patient was discharged, the volunteers of an 'after-care committee' would keep an eye on him and report back to Ranchi. Every six months the hospital sent out a 'welfare inquiry' letter, to which former patients and their families would reply.

The staff went through a transition as well. To begin with, all male attendants were replaced with qualified nurses. Every nurse had to clear a written exam before her appointment was confirmed. She was to later obtain a certificate of proficiency in mental nursing. Practical training at Ranchi came to be accredited in Britain for this certificate, just as it was for the postgraduate diploma in psychological medicine. There were regular lectures at the hospital for doctors as well as nurses. At a weekly meeting, they discussed the clinical history, diagnosis, treatment and prognosis of new patients. Patients were invited to staff conferences to give their views on how things were going, and on new things being planned.

Dr Berkeley-Hill did not confine his ideas to the institution that he ran. A prolific writer, he contributed to various newspapers and journals. He also addressed a large number of scientific, medical, social, and religious gatherings. One of his concerns was that the medical profession in Britain and British India did not pay enough attention to the psychological roots of mental disorders. He believed that doctors must have a basic understanding of human psychology. A trained psychoanalyst himself, Dr Berkeley-Hill underlined the benefits of psychotherapy. He also argued the case for psychiatric treatment outside mental hospitals. In his view, an outpatient clinic would enable people to seek treatment at an early stage of illness, and for disorders that were relatively less disabling. And apart from building public confidence, these clinics would give psychiatry a place in mainstream medicine.

Although Ranchi was privileged and Dr Berkeley-Hill was persuasive, this did not mean that he always got his way. Much to his annoyance, some of his ideas were shot down, and others were abandoned once he retired. But very many of them would prevail.

~

In 1913, there were 264 'idiots' and 58 'imbeciles' in the mental hospitals of British India. What did these labels mean? Both implied an incurable learning disability, from birth or from an early age. Being severely disabled, an 'idiot' could not protect himself from common physical dangers. While an 'imbecile' was relatively less disabled, he could neither look after his affairs nor himself. 'Idiots' and 'imbeciles' thus needed special care.

That same year, Britain passed a law on the education, training, and care of 'mental defectives'. This law dealt with public and private services, for children and adults, at their home and in institutions. In British India, however, no such law existed. 'Mental defectives' were covered by the same law as the mentally ill. On the orders of a magistrate, they too could be admitted to a mental hospital by relatives, or by the police. Some were sent to jail, possibly on trivial charges, before they might be transferred to a mental hospital. As they could never be fit to stand trial, they would spend the rest of their lives as 'criminal insanes'.

In February 1925, the matter of 'mental defectives' cropped up in the Council of States – the upper house of British India's legislature. Ebrahim Haroon Jaffer moved a resolution that provincial governments be asked to investigate the best means of 'dealing quickly and adequately with cases of mental defectives, particularly of the minor and curable kind'. This led to a brief, and somewhat confused discussion. Speaking for the Government of India, home secretary J. Crerar assured members that it took a 'very serious and sympathetic view' of the matter. He pointed to the lack of 'accurate, reliable, practical data', and the need for 'practical and constructive suggestions'. Even so, since 'mental deficiency' was a provincial subject, the Government of India could not interfere. The most it could do was to circulate the council's proceedings to local governments, and convey the 'deep sympathy' that it felt. With no choice but to accept this outcome, Jaffer withdrew his resolution.

The next year, Dr Berkeley-Hill came up with a plan. He proposed an annexe to the Ranchi hospital, where 'mentally defective' children would be taught basic skills. These children would be admitted directly, that is, without going through the legal system. Over a span of nine months, Dr Berkeley-Hill's proposal travelled from the board of trustees to the Bihar and Orissa government, and onward to the other local governments that funded the European mental hospital at Ranchi. None of the governments agreed.

Not one to be deterred, Dr Berkeley-Hill gave up on direct admission, but went ahead with the idea of special training. He engaged a lady teacher to start a class 'somewhat on the lines of the Montessori system'. And though she was new to this sort of work, he reported that the results were 'not at all unsatisfactory'.

Madras managed to inch ahead of Ranchi – albeit very, very slowly. In 1925, Dr Hensman had come up with a plan for a small home for 'mental defectives' as an annexe to the Madras mental hospital. The provincial government was open to the idea, and even invited Dr Berkeley-Hill to Madras for consultation. But citing 'financial stringency', it did nothing else for over a decade.

The idea was revived in 1937. To begin with, a small cottage was converted into a training centre for boys. Here they were taught through pictures, stories, drawing, games, singing, dancing, and the odd excursion. The boys also learned spinning, weaving, and carpentry. The original plan for a separate children's home had to wait a while longer. Thanks to a private benefactor, Sri M. Rungayya Chetty, it was finally inaugurated in 1941. The home was less than ideal. It was, for instance, rather small, and it did not take in girls. But despite these drawbacks, it was the only public facility of its kind in the country.

For several decades, 'mental defectives' would continue to be admitted to mental hospitals. But in 1993, a new mental health law came into force. This would not apply to 'mental defectives'. Two years passed. A separate law for 'disabled persons' – including the 'mentally retarded' – was finally enacted in 1995.

~

Left, as they were, to their own devices, the alienists had a rather lonely job. There were few opportunities to compare notes with specialists in other parts of the country. This would change when the Indian branch of the Royal Medico-Psychological Association was set up in 1939. The association held its first conference at the Lahore mental hospital that year. The move had come too late for the early alienists. But it was to become a source of support and solidarity for those who followed in their tracks.

> Our gathering together here to-day for the first conference of alienists ever held in India is an encouraging indication of our unity of purpose ... Bound together by a common purpose, we must not remain merely smouldering faggots[10]. Let us become flaming torches to spread psychiatric enlightenment throughout the length and breadth of this great sub-continent, until we kindle a beacon whose rays will spread light and warmth where there has hitherto been nothing but desolation and wintry darkness.[11]

---

[10] An obsolete term for people who speak loudly.

[11] C. J. Lodge Patch, 'A Century of Psychiatry in the Punjab', *The Journal of Mental Science*, vol. 85, no. 356 (May 1939): 391.

SIX

Trends in Treatment

The reason why Hospital treatment is very desirable and most soothing in many mental disorders is that the trained staff of the Hospital know how to approach the patient properly[,] and the patient feels that at last he is understood and has some one to rely upon[;] and by making the most of his confidence[,] it is often possible to avoid many difficulties and eventually to lead him back to mental health. As usual[,] strict watch was kept over the latest mental and medical journals for anything likely to influence in a direct or indirect way the course of the malady[;] and neither expense nor trouble is ever allowed to stand in the way of the employment of the latest discoveries if thereby the patient can in any way be benefited.[12]

Medieval times saw insanity as a mysterious malady that was brought on by occult or evil forces. Those whom it afflicted seemed to behave in a bizarre manner that defied reason. They could be disturbing and disruptive, even dangerous. So institutions were created where the insane could be confined and controlled. But

---

[12] J.E. Dhunjibhoy, *Annual Report on the Working of the Ranchi Indian Mental Hospital, Kanke, in Bihar and Orissa, for the Year 1934* (Patna: Superintendent, Government Printing, Bihar and Orissa, 1935), 11.

by the middle of the 19th century, these notions were being overturned. The malady was seen as an illness – like a host of other illnesses – whose origin was to be found in the human body. The 'modern' view called for a humane and therapeutic environment for those who were mentally ill.

As this view took root in Britain, asylums began to be refashioned as mental hospitals. The change in course veered away from confinement and control of the mentally ill. Instead, it prescribed liberty, occupation, recreation, exercise, and entertainment. In principle, mental hospitals in British India were expected to follow the example being set 'at home'. In practice, few of them did, and only in a modest way. But in the new era, the mental hospitals run by alienists were expected to do much more, and much better.

~

Ranchi was the first to liberate its patients from curbs in everyday life. Soon after the hospital opened, it put a stop to the use of restraints and seclusion. By 1935, it had taken the radical step of removing locks and bolts from the doors of all wards. This meant that patients were never locked in, whether by day or by night. They were free to roam the premises as and when they wished. From 1937, they no longer had to wear the ready-made clothes that were handed out by the hospital. Instead, they could choose the fabric and design of outfits that would then be tailored to their measurements. If they liked, their clothes could even be brought over from home. A small shop was opened on the campus, where patients could buy various things for themselves. In another first, Ranchi did away with the strict segregation of the sexes. While men and women resided in separate sections of the hospital, they came together for common activities during the day. All patients who were fit to work were supposed to attend occupational therapy each morning. But they were offered a large variety of choices, and were free to pick the ones they liked.

During their stay at Ranchi, patients remained connected with the outside world. In the early years, 'dependable' patients were allowed to go for walks outside the premises – without an escort. By 1925, virtually all patients were eligible for this privilege. Women, however, were normally accompanied by an ayah. As patients preferred to patronise the local market, the shop on the campus was closed down. Patients were free to write and receive as many letters as they wished. Most of these were uncensored. And visitors could drop in to see them during working hours on any day of the week. Once a patient had improved enough to be considered for discharge, he could be sent home for a period of two months. If that went well, he would then be formally discharged. This system of 'parole' – or leave of absence – had been put in place as early as 1922.

Little is known about the degree of freedom at the other hospitals, but efforts were certainly being made. In the absence of an alienist at Lahore since the outbreak of World War I, a large number of patients were being kept in mechanical restraints. And all patients were being routinely locked up for much of the day. With the return of an alienist in 1922, these practices came to a halt. Yeravda had its own shop where patients could buy 'such things as cigarettes, biddies, fruit, sweets, writing paper, soaps, ribbons, etc., etc.'. Taking a cue from Ranchi, select patients were allowed to go out for walks on their own at Kanke, Lahore, and Madras. Kanke also organised shopping expeditions to the markets in town. Its patients had a say in the kind of occupational therapy that they took up. Some needed to be persuaded to work, but the staff was forbidden to compel them to do so. From 1937, Kanke too began to send patients home on leave of absence before taking a final call on their discharge.

Did the other hospitals go as far as Ranchi did? Probably not. Liberty came at a cost that a crowded, poorly staffed hospital was less likely to afford. Besides, liberty also came with risks – of a misdemeanour, a lapse, an accident, an escape. Even if an alienist was willing to take chances, the local government might not approve.

The hospitals tried to keep their patients busy in what they saw as occupational therapy. Except for those who were sick or infirm, most patients were capable of some kind of work. And many were capable of learning new skills. But it was not always easy to come up with suitable occupations on a sizeable scale.

One option was for patients to help the staff in the infirmary, wards, kitchen, stores, office, or library. Another was for them to assist the hospital's tailor, mechanic, carpenter, blacksmith, mason, and so on. Some patients at Kanke, Lahore, Madras, Nagpur, Tezpur, and Yeravda were engaged in this kind of work. But hospitals would have to find other ways to keep hundreds of patients busy.

They did not have to look very far. Each had land that was arable, or else could be made arable. Except Ranchi, all of them introduced farming as a form of occupational therapy. Its benefits were many. Farming provided plenty of outdoor exercise. An assortment of tasks – from light to heavy – could be assigned to patients according to their ability. While those from rural areas were already familiar with the work, others could take to it too. And fresh produce from the farm was a welcome addition to the patients' meals. In 1930, Kanke had engaged 140 patients in farming. Ten years later, the number shot up to as many as 500. In a good year, the farm would meet most of the hospital's requirement of vegetables and fruits. And sometimes it even yielded a surplus for sale.

Other kinds of work demanded a different set of skills. Weaving was introduced in all hospitals. Lahore, Madras, and Tezpur often got by with fabric woven by their own patients. Much of Lahore's supply of blankets was produced in-house. Articles such as rugs, mats, brooms, and baskets were crafted in several hospitals. And sewing, knitting, and embroidery were common pursuits. While the items made by patients were chiefly put to daily use, the surplus – if any – was sold in the market. At Lahore, for instance, the sale of munj mats often earned a tidy sum. At Madras, a few patients were taught to make soap and hand-made paper in 1946. Other than this, the introduction of non-traditional activities was rather rare. For very many years, Yeravda had been keen to engage more of its patients in skilled tasks – particularly as its European and Parsi patients were not given to manual work. But the lack of instructors and suitable premises had held it back. A weaving shed and a carpenter's workshop would finally open in the year 1939. Tezpur had reported that the 'better class' of patients 'loathed' working on the land. In the absence of instructors, neither Tezpur nor Nagpur was able to step up skilled activities.

At a time when other hospitals were engaging their patients in useful work, Ranchi decided to differ. It brought in professional occupational therapists to guide patients in a variety of appealing activities. The list included skilled work, like boot-making, book-binding, and carpentry. It also had assorted crafts, such as making artificial flowers, embroidery, clay modelling, and papier mâché. Articles made by patients would be put up for exhibition as well as for sale. But the utility or saleability of these articles was seen as purely incidental. In 1934, there was a change in leadership at Ranchi. With this came a change in the idea of occupational therapy. In the new dispensation, this therapy was meant to be 'constructive' rather than 'fancy'. The focus of occupational therapy thus shifted to the kind of work that was of practical use at the hospital.

Was occupational therapy pushed as a means to raise revenue for the government? This did not seem to be the case. The income that it earned was neither steady nor substantial. But it did seem that this therapy was expected to pay for itself – in monetary rather than medical terms. In general, work that saved on hospital expenses was preferred, whether or not more therapeutic options could be found.

Avenues for recreation and exercise were in plenty at Kanke, Madras, Ranchi, and Yeravda. Football, cricket, hockey, tennis, and badminton were among the popular outdoor games. Women played badminton and tennis at Kanke as well as Yeravda. Ranchi introduced mixed teams for hockey and basketball, and 'ladies' vs 'gents' hockey matches. When Madras put together a cricket team in 1914, it was the first to venture into competitive sports. All four hospitals played friendly matches against outside teams – home and away – and also took part in tournaments. At Madras, patients competed in the annual events hosted by the South Indian Athletic Association. Ranchi arranged for swimming and rowing in a nearby lake through the summer months. And 'musical drill' was a regular feature on winter mornings. Patients could play table tennis at Kanke and Madras, and billiards at Madras and Yeravda. The calendar of all four hospitals was marked by regular walks, rambles, drives, and picnics.

Other hospitals too offered recreation to their patients, though this may not have been as varied or as frequent. At Agra, for instance, only the 'better class' of patients engaged in regular walks, football, and tennis. Tezpur did not have a vehicle to take patients for outings. Apparently, patients at Lahore could not be induced to take part in outdoor games. But some of them had a great interest in birds and animals. Deer, rabbits, guinea-pigs, fowls, peafowl, parrots, and pigeons that roamed the hospital gardens were cared for by these patients – and at times, trained by them as well. There was even the curious case of a 'criminal lunatic' who had taught his pet cat and pigeon to live 'in the greatest harmony'.

Board games, gramophones, books, magazines, and newspapers were the usual sources of entertainment. In addition, the hospitals hosted performances by musicians, dancers, theatre troupes, magicians, comedians, jugglers, puppeteers, and sundry other artistes. Kanke, Ranchi and Yeravda had a cinema projector and screened films every week. Film shows at Yeravda stopped in 1932, when talkies took over from the era of silent films. After that, small groups of 'well-behaved' patients would be gifted free passes by philanthropic theatre owners. A similar arrangement was in place at Lahore, Madras, and Nagpur. Through the summer months, a 'moonlight promenade concert' was held at Ranchi on Mondays. The weekly 'social' at Ranchi and Yeravda would be accompanied either by gramophone music or by a live band. Ranchi had its own band, and so did Kanke. Besides performing solo each week, their bands also played at get-togethers, games, and picnics. An outside band came over once a month at Madras and at Yeravda. Ranchi's patients took to the stage themselves, with performances of music, dance, theatre, and gymnastics.

As a rule, the hospitals celebrated important festivals with special entertainment and special meals or 'treats'. On a more spiritual note, Kanke, Madras, and Ranchi arranged for devotional singing, discourses, and prayers on a regular basis.

Many pleasures in the lives of patients were gifts from public-spirited persons. Books, newspaper subscriptions, and cinema passes came in. An artiste might perform free of charge for the patients. And a donor might sponsor an outing or a 'treat'. Contributions could take different shapes and sizes. Lahore, for instance, bought a motor bus and a cinema projector thanks to generous donations from Sir Edward Maclagan, then Governor of Punjab, the Maharaja of Faridkot, and the Maharaja of Patiala. Mr Jamal Muhi-ud-din presented Madras with a motor bus. A group of lady volunteers faithfully visited the hospital to spend time with the women and involve them in needlework, games, and drama.

Yeravda was blessed with very many benefactors. Mr A.C. Patel gifted the hospital with a cinema projector. He arranged for free theatre tickets. He contributed towards musical instruments. He sponsored picnics. He was even a regular figure at the patients' weekly entertainment and monthly dance. For several years, Mr Mody of the Empire Cinema Company sent his assistants to screen films at the hospital every week. Trustees of the late Mr M.N. Wadia funded the construction of a tennis court, and the purchase of a billiards table. Yeravda received four pianos as gifts. Two were from a Parsi gentleman who wished to remain anonymous. A Fiat motor bus came from the Bombay Women Presidency Council, and a Citroen bus from the Sanj Vartaman Ambulance Bus Fund. A rowboat and a radio set were among Yeravda's many prized presents.

There is no doubt that liberty, occupation, recreation, exercise, and entertainment made for a more humane environment for the mentally ill. But were they also therapeutic? According to the alienists, they certainly were.

By 1933, alienists were in charge at Agra, Kanke, Lahore, Madras, Nagpur, Ranchi, Tezpur, and Yeravda. Over the years, each hospital had introduced its own set of therapies – in its own way and at its own pace. At no two hospitals were these identical.

Even as the same therapy could differ across hospitals, it could also differentiate between patients. Had cost not been a chronic concern, it may have been possible to benefit many more patients in many more ways.

~

Discoveries during the early 20th century began to change the way mental illness was understood, identified, and treated. Drawn from the science of physiology as well as psychology, the ideas that surfaced were by no means definitive. They would be challenged and debated across the world.

Systems to classify mental disorders were revised, and methods of diagnosis were refined. Standards for both would, however, vary from one country to another. In the past, doctors would attempt to tackle the most striking symptom that they saw. Now they were more likely to look at a range of symptoms, and at patterns that showed up over time.

Since medical science could not yet explain the cause of most mental disorders, the search for solutions still lacked a rational basis. Even so, the early results of experiments were reported in reputed medical journals. As these were tested at different locations, a variety of protocols and procedures emerged. Promising therapies quickly found their way into mental hospitals and clinics across Europe and America. None was backed by solid evidence at the time. And many were associated with serious risk. Yet they seemed to offer new hope to the mentally ill – for reprieve and for recovery.

~

Back in India, the alienists picked up the latest findings on foreign visits and from foreign journals. These they then adapted through a process of trial and error. From the 1920s to the 1940s, at least a dozen new therapies were tried at different hospitals at different points in time. Opinion on certain treatments was divided. For example, Ranchi decided to limit the use of insulin coma therapy. On the other hand, Lahore, Madras, and Yeravda seemed to have fewer reservations. Sulfosin therapy was favoured at Kanke, but was not particularly popular elsewhere. While Ranchi and Kanke used narcoanalysis and prolonged sleep therapy, Lahore was the only other hospital to mention these methods. Some treatments had few takers. Psychotherapy, for instance, was only cited – and briefly – in reports from Kanke, Nagpur, and Ranchi. None of the mental hospitals in British India recommended the surgical procedure of prefrontal leucotomy. But several patients at the Bangalore mental hospital were taken to the Krishna Rajendra Hospital, Mysore, for this surgery.

Four treatments met with a fair amount of approval at several mental hospitals in the country. These were hydrotherapy, insulin coma therapy, cardiazol therapy, and electroconvulsive therapy.

Hydrotherapy was a standard treatment in the West long before it came to India. One of its forms – the prolonged bath – was introduced at Ranchi in 1921, and at Kanke in 1926. This 'soothing and pleasant' method was found useful in restlessness, excitement, and insomnia, and its effect on psychotic patients could be 'astonishing'. The patient was to remain immersed for several hours in a specially designed tub. There was a steady inflow of warm water of a specified temperature, which drained out continuously. The bath would be repeated over weeks, if not months. Some patients at Ranchi clocked over 450 hours of hydrotherapy. More than 1,800 patients at Kanke received this treatment during the 1930s. Hydrotherapy was also introduced at Madras in 1928, Tezpur in 1933, Nagpur in 1935, and Agra in 1939.

A new treatment for schizophrenia was announced by Polish psychiatrist Manfred Sakel in 1933. It used insulin to induce a state of coma, from which the patient was later revived with the help of glucose. Constant monitoring was necessary, as there was a danger of the patient slipping into an irreversible coma. The procedure would be repeated at least a couple of times a week, over a period of about six weeks. Insulin coma therapy caught on in the West, and encouraging results were reported from various places. It was tried at Lahore, Madras, Nagpur, Ranchi, and at Yeravda.

After Hungarian psychiatrist Ladislas Meduna published his results with the synthetic drug cardiazol in 1935, this therapy was widely recommended in cases of schizophrenia. Later, it was also found useful for patients with mood disorders. A typical case involved about 20 sessions over a period of two months or so. Each session started with a calibrated dose of the drug, which was administered by intravenous injection. This would cause a severe convulsion almost immediately, which usually lasted less than a minute. The patient would then lose consciousness for about half an hour. Following a period of rest, he would generally be up and about by the end of the day. Cardiazol therapy was commonly regarded as both simple as well as safe. However, a patient might experience extreme fear while the drug was taking effect. Unless proper precautions were taken, he could also dislocate a joint or fracture a vertebra during a convulsion. In due course, the method was introduced at Kanke, Lahore, Madras, Nagpur, Ranchi, and Yeravda. An account of its early experience at Kanke was published in *The Lancet* and *The Indian Medical Gazette* in 1938.

The fourth method also involved induced convulsions. But

here they were brought on by an electrical current, not by a drug. Electroconvulsive treatment was devised by Italian psychiatrists Ugo Cerletti and Lucio Bini in 1938. Widely accepted in several countries, it was used to treat schizophrenia, mood disorders, and psychoneuroses. The treatment involved passing a mild electric current through the patient's brain for a fraction of a second. The patient would instantly lose consciousness, and experience a major seizure. In a few minutes, he would become conscious and have no recollection of the procedure. The treatment could be repeated a couple of times a week, and last for as many as a dozen sessions. It was generally seen as quick, easy, and inexpensive. But it did carry the risk of permanent memory loss. Even so, electroconvulsive therapy was considered superior to insulin coma therapy, as well as to drug-induced convulsion therapies. It was adopted at Agra, Kanke, Lahore, Madras, Nagpur, Ranchi, and Yervada.

Did the experimental therapies actually work? According to the alienists, they did help in certain cases. While the older lines of treatment were generic, the newer ones were prescribed for an individual patient. Aside from close personal attention, they called for specialised medical knowledge, skills, and facilities. These therapies would place new demands on alienists, physicians, nurses, and attendants. And before long, they would call into question the norms by which mental hospitals were staffed, equipped, and funded.

~

Through much of the 19th century, the best that psychological medicine had to offer was little other than nutrition, rest, hygiene, pleasant surroundings, and attention to 'physical' ailments.

But by the middle of the 20th century, it advised generic treatment – such as liberty, occupation, recreation, exercise, and entertainment – as well as special individual treatment, like hydrotherapy, insulin coma therapy, cardiazol therapy, and electroconvulsive therapy. The newer lines of treatment had not yet been scientifically proven. In the years to come, many would be disputed, discredited, and discarded. And the search for more effective, safe, and ethical choices would go on.

[T]here has been a great awakening in India, in Psychiatry as in the other branches of medicine. This awakening has destroyed smug-complacency and callous indifference to the fate of mental patients. People have begun to realize that psychiatry is an important branch of medicine, that the lunatic asylum has evolved into the modern mental hospital, and that the insane individual who used to be put away for safe-keeping has been transformed into a patient undergoing systematic scientific treatment. But compared to the progress made in America and England, India has a long distance yet to travel.[13]

---

[13] M.V. Govindaswamy, 'Mental Disorder in India – a Review and a Prospect', *The Indian Journal of Social Work*, vol. 7, no. 1 (1946): 42.

SEVEN

Legacy of the Raj

Finally, I would stress that the conditions in some of the Mental Hospitals in India today are disgraceful, and have the makings of a major public scandal.[14]

The history of lunatic asylums in colonial India has been written by scholars from different schools of thought. As a result, the asylum has been analysed from all sorts of angles. Did it, for instance, originate as a place to hide 'abnormal' white people from 'native' eyes? Was it an instrument of racial subjugation? Of social oppression? Of stifling subversion and dissent? Of maintaining public order? Did it seek to profit from the labour of its inmates? How did it deal with caste, class, and gender? And why did it lag so far behind medical advances in the empire, and in the colony?

Very little has been said about asylum reforms that began in the early 20th century. How did the 'new era' pan out over the last stretch of colonial rule? And what did it hold for the treatment and care of the mentally ill? While scholars are yet to

---

[14] Colonel M. Taylor's account of his tour of mental hospitals, *Report of the Health Survey and Development Committee, volume III: Appendices* (Delhi: Manager of Publications, Government of India, 1946): 74.

delve deep into these questions, there are enough clues that point to preliminary answers.

~

The 'new era' was a much delayed response to the modern notion that insanity was an illness that called for humane and therapeutic treatment. Most asylums in British India were till then under part-time superintendents who were general medical practitioners. If they were to be managed on scientific lines, they would have to be run by full-time specialists. The Government of India thus went in for six large mental hospitals, each to be headed by an alienist. By 1925, alienists were in charge at Agra, Kanke, Lahore, Madras, Ranchi, and at Yeravda.

The plan was to gradually replace small mental hospitals with large ones that were better designed, and better run. This may well have happened, but for a shake up in the administration. In 1919, the central government had transferred several of its powers – including the management of mental hospitals – to provincial governments. From this point on, the central government had merely an advisory role in the matter. While it did advise provincial governments to upgrade its small mental hospitals, the response was tepid at best. No old hospital was shut, and no new hospital was opened. Instead, extra wards were added from time to time. In due course, the hospitals at Nagpur and Tezpur grew large enough to require a full-time superintendent. Fortunately, both were to get the services of an alienist.

The success of the 'new era' relied entirely on the alienists. In the early years, such officers were in short supply. It was hard to find a substitute when one was on long leave. And it was hard to find a replacement when one of them retired. So, every now and

                    Daman Singh

then, a non-alienist would take over for varying lengths of time. Such periods were very long when Britain was at war.

During World War I, the post of superintendent had changed hands often, and did not always remain a full-time job. Even though the war ended in 1918, it took a while for medical services to return to normal. The tenure of alienists was thus disrupted from 1914 to 1921 at Yeravda, from 1915 to 1924 at Madras, from 1915 to 1919 at Agra, from 1916 to 1922 at Lahore, from 1918 to 1923 at Berhampore, and from 1918 to 1919 at Ranchi. After two decades of peace, World War II broke out in 1939. Once again, there was a massive mobilisation of medical personnel. Agra, Kanke, Lahore, Madras, and Yeravda were without an alienist for much of the war.

The two world wars were fought for about ten years in all. But they obstructed the progress of the alienists for much longer.

Where did the alienists stand on the treatment of mental disorders? By the 1940s, there was some consensus on the subject. The alienists stressed the importance of nutrition, rest, hygiene, pleasant surroundings, and attention to 'physical' ailments. Their prescription included generic treatment – such as liberty, occupation, recreation, exercise, and entertainment – as well as special individual treatment, like hydrotherapy, insulin coma therapy, cardiazol therapy, and electroconvulsive therapy.

As each hospital reported to a different authority, facilities for treatment were bound to vary. Even so, a range of therapies was available to some – if not all – patients at Agra, Kanke, Lahore, Madras, Nagpur, Ranchi, Tezpur, and Yervada. Several hospitals would face unexpected hurdles when various supplies were blocked during World War II. Yervada, for instance, had to close down its weaving shed and carpentry workshop, as raw material could not be sourced. Hydrotherapy stopped at Tezpur since the equipment could neither be repaired nor replaced.

Nagpur was unable to procure cardiazol. And the arrival of apparatus for electroconvulsive treatment at Kanke and Ranchi was excessively delayed. Lahore even found that it could not buy blankets and clothing 'owing to war'.

The 'new era' had introduced the idea of a modern mental hospital to British India. Bit by bit, this idea found a foothold in the eight large hospitals that were led by alienists. Every alienist was a trained specialist in the field of psychological medicine. But each hospital had emerged at a different point in time. Each had evolved independently. And each was accountable to a separate government agency. As a result, the gains achieved at one hospital were seldom shared by the other seven.

Meanwhile, small mental hospitals had continued to exist. In 1933, there were nine such hospitals. These accounted for a quarter of the total capacity of all mental hospitals in the colony. Some may have picked up tips from the more modern ones. But since none was run by a full-time superintendent, let alone an alienist, that was not very likely.

Without a unified policy on mental hospitals, the progress of the 'new era' was destined to be fragmented. While it ushered in new methods for the treatment and care of mental illness, it also allowed old methods to remain pretty much unchanged.

⁓

What did the 'new era' offer to those who were mentally ill?

In the year 1900, the 23 mental hospitals in British India could accommodate no more than 5,413 patients. By 1925, their number had dropped to 17, but their capacity grew to 7,304 persons. While no new hospitals were then added, the existing ones continued to expand. As of 1946, the 17 mental hospitals could thus take in 9,699 patients.

The 17 hospitals were not evenly distributed across provinces. Bengal and Orissa, for instance, had none. Their patients had to be sent to Bihar. Bengal also took the liberty of keeping some patients in Calcutta's central jail. The North-West Frontier Province did not have a hospital either. Its patients were kept in prison at Peshawar. And all the provinces, barring Bombay, were known to put persons in jail while their mental state was being assessed

Several hospitals often complained that they were short of accommodation. At the close of 1946, Bombay province had 26 per cent more patients than beds. In Madras province the figure was even higher at 57 per cent. The most crowded hospital was in Madras city, with an alarming 78 per cent of patients over and above its sanctioned strength. This was despite the fact that around 300 former jail inmates had been recently transported some 150 kilometres to the Cuddalore jail. Elsewhere, overcrowding might be confined to a certain part of the year, or to a certain section of the hospital. Kanke had a policy of not admitting patients beyond its capacity. As it was usually full, private patients were simply turned away, while others were sent to the Hazaribagh jail to wait it out.

In truth, the colony was grossly short of medical facilities for the mentally ill. And it had been so for years.

What do we know about the men and women who were admitted to these mental hospitals? Unfortunately, nothing very much. They came from all parts of the country. They were of all races, all classes, all faiths, and all ages. They may have come from jail, from the streets, or from home. In official parlance, they would thus be labelled as 'criminal insanes', 'paupers', or private patients. Among these categories, the number of private patients was relatively low.

A mental hospital was generally the last resort for a private patient. It was customary to first turn to the occult, to faith, and to traditional methods of healing. When all else failed, as it may have often done, the mental hospital was the only option that remained. Even so, this option was not exactly popular. As a matter of fact, Indians had taken to Western medicine in a pretty big way. After a century of colonial rule, there were 7,652 hospitals and dispensaries in British India. And of its 47,400 registered medical practitioners, as many as 73 percent were engaged in private practice. Why then did the local population not take to psychological medicine?

The alienists came up with several reasons for this. To begin with, the public was ill-informed about the early signs of mental illness, and about the value of early treatment. This was not surprising – so was the general medical practitioner. Consequently, only a severely ill person was likely to be referred to a mental hospital. But a mental hospital was not accessible to all. And admission was not easy either. Once admitted, a patient would disappear behind closed doors. There was no saying how he would be treated, or when he could come out. And his entire family would be tainted by the stigma of mental illness.

The solutions suggested by the alienists were by no means simple. The public had to be enlightened. The medical fraternity had to be educated. Mental hospitals had to be set up at many more locations. They had to open their doors just as other hospitals did. Admission procedures had to be simplified. And psychological medicine had to find a place for itself outside mental hospitals.

By the 1930s, a number of therapies had been found suitable for outpatients. Some were useful in treating early mental illness, while others were of benefit in an advanced stage of illness. During World War II, Ranchi had offered outpatient services to European and Indian military personnel. Other than this purely temporary arrangement, no public mental hospital in British India had treated outpatients. But Lumbini Park Mental Hospital, a small private facility in Calcutta, did. And so did the two mental hospitals in the princely states of Mysore and Travancore.

Treatment of mental illness was no longer the sole preserve of the mental hospital. Fledgling outpatient clinics had opened at a few general hospitals and medical colleges, both public as well as private. Three were in Bombay alone – at Sir Jamsetjee Jeejebhoy Hospital, St. George's Hospital, and King Edward Memorial Hospital. Calcutta had one at Carmichael Medical College and another at Medical College Hospital. Clinics also ran at Rayapuram Hospital in Madras, Prince of Wales Medical College Hospital in Patna, King George Medical College Hospital in Lucknow, and at King George Hospital at Vizagapatam. And the very first 'child guidance clinic' was started by Sir Dorabji Tata Institute of Social Sciences in Bombay.

One day, the outpatient clinic would open up immense possibilities. It would bring treatment within easy reach of those who were in need. It would not ask that patients be certified as insane by the law. And it would help to lessen the fear, prejudice, and superstition surrounding mental illness. That day, however, was a very long way off.

~

In 1943, when the days of colonial rule were clearly numbered, the Government of India set up a committee to chalk out a plan to rebuild the health sector after the war. Over the next two years, this committee studied official records, it sought the views of experts from India and abroad, it travelled, and it deliberated. Chaired by Sir Joseph Bhore, the Health Survey and

Development Committee came out with a three-volume report in 1946.

The report brought out the huge contrast between Britain and British India. Infant mortality in England and Wales was 58 per thousand live births. In British India the figure was 162. Life expectancy in England and Wales was 59 years for men and 63 years for women. In British India it was 27 years for both. The death rate in England and Wales was 12.4 per thousand. In British India it was 22.4 per thousand – and at least half these deaths were preventable.

The Bhore committee decided that medical services in British India were 'altogether inadequate'. There were simply not enough hospitals, dispensaries, doctors, and nurses. In England and Wales the ratio of hospital beds to the population was 1:300. In British India the ratio was 1:4,000. Not surprisingly, there was 'considerable' overcrowding in wards. The quality of medical service too left 'much to be desired'. At one dispensary, the committee observed that the average time given to a patient was about a minute. It was only 48 seconds at another.

The state of mental health services was even worse. In the absence of estimates for the incidence of mental illness, the report assumed that two per thousand persons needed hospital care. It also assumed that four per thousand persons were mentally deficient. This would translate into about 800,000 mentally ill, and 1,600,000 mentally deficient persons. Yet there were no more than 10,000 beds in mental hospitals in the entire country. The functioning of these hospitals was 'far from satisfactory'. They lacked trained professionals and were 'disgracefully understaffed'. Few were in a position to offer specialised therapy to patients. And few were equipped to provide specialised training.

The Bhore committee was of the view that recent progress

in understanding and treating mental disorder had been 'so spectacular' that the chances of recovery were actually better than in other illnesses. With inputs from specialists from different parts of the country, it proposed a country-wide mental health programme. The contours of this programme would have to be based on the needs of the provinces. While it would take some time to determine these needs, various steps could be taken immediately.

Noting that 'mental' and 'physical' health were closely related, the committee suggested that the health establishment – central and provincial – have a branch dealing with mental health. The existing mental hospitals would have to be radically improved to bring them up to modern standards. And there was a need to build seven new hospitals. The plan was to quadruple the total number of beds over the next ten years. Ultimately, it was advisable to dedicate certain hospitals solely to the treatment of mental illness. Others would be better suited as homes for the care of incurable patients, or as homes for the care of mentally deficient persons.

An intensive effort would be required to train specialists for administrative and clinical posts. Ideally, these officers should have a postgraduate degree in general medicine, as well as a diploma in psychological medicine. Universities in provincial capitals needed to offer suitable courses for this diploma. In the meantime, it was advisable to train 40 doctors abroad over the next ten years. The committee also identified places to train occupational therapists, psychiatric social workers, psychologists, nurses, and attendants.

The report of the Health Survey and Development Committee was an authoritative document. But it had been placed in the hands of a regime that was on its way out. In the years that followed, it would serve as a guide to successive central and provincial governments. Each government would pick and choose what fitted in with its priorities.

~

India became independent on 15 August 1947. So did Pakistan, a separate country carved out of the subcontinent. The struggle for freedom had been remarkably peaceful, but the process of partition was shockingly violent. Whether by hook or by crook, the princely states acceded to either of the two dominions. On 26 January 1950, India declared itself a democratic republic. Its new constitution resolved to secure justice, liberty, and equality for all citizens.

What would this mean for citizens who happened to be mentally ill?

> The aftermath of Indian Independence might well be – but must not be permitted to be – followed by disillusionment. Disillusionment, frustration, futility, lack of economic and emotional security, find their vent in mass hysteria, labour strikes, disorganisation in society and of family life, and destruction of old loyalties and traditions and of individual and group morale. These are larger problems of mental health to combat in which the individual and the state should come together in closer co-operation.[15]

---

[15] M.V. Govindaswamy, 'Mental Disorder in India – a Review and a Prospect (Since 1946)', *Indian Journal of Social Work*, vol. 9, no. 2 (1948): 100.

PART TWO

EIGHT

Lahore

This has been a very difficult and unfortunate year for the Punjab Mental Hospital.[16]

In March 1946, Britain had begun discussions with Indian political parties on the transfer of power to a government of independent India. But it did not take long for the idea of an undivided India to fall apart. The movement for a separate nation where Muslims would be in a majority gained ground in the months that followed. Savage communal riots broke out in Bengal in August. They spread to Bihar in September and the North-West Frontier Province in December, before engulfing Punjab in March 1947. On 3 June 1947, the plan to divide the country on religious lines was announced. The frontiers between the two new nations were yet to be drawn. But wherever they would lie, people were expected to continue to live where they did. That did not happen. Even before an independent Pakistan and India came into being on the midnight of 14 and 15 August 1947, thousands of people had fled their homes. After partition,

---

[16] *Annual Report on the Working of the West Punjab Mental Hospital, Lahore, 1947* (Lahore: Superintendent, Government Printing, West Punjab, 1949), 3.

India was flanked by Pakistan on the east as well as the west. Over 12 million people would cross its borders that year.

The wave of migration in the west took place amidst gruesome killing, rape, abduction, arson, and looting. Once the border was in place, the two governments had stepped in to evacuate their respective citizens in foot convoys, in trucks, in trains, and even in planes. By the end of 1947, Muslims from various parts of India had been escorted to West Pakistan. And by April 1948, Hindus and Sikhs from West Punjab, the North-West Frontier Province, and Bahawalpur had been escorted to India. The evacuation from Sind had, however, carried on right through the year.

These operations did not include citizens who were in mental hospitals at the time.

~

As Punjab province was divided between Pakistan and India, its assets were divided between West Punjab and East Punjab. A number of provincial institutions were supposed to cater to both halves for a while. For instance, the university in Lahore – a city that went to West Punjab – was to continue to serve East Punjab for a year. Similarly, the mental hospital at Lahore was to serve East Punjab for the next three years. Later, both these decisions would be reversed. East Punjab moved quickly to create its own university, albeit without a campus, in October 1947. It also moved to set up its own mental hospital, but this would take much longer.

Lahore had witnessed bursts of violence since early March that year. These pushed many Hindus and Sikhs to head eastward. But the exodus only began when the entire city was ravaged by riots in August. Amidst the turbulence in Lahore, the mental hospital had apparently escaped harm. It had posted its own guards and patrols in the premises, within which non-Muslim staff and their families were told to remain. But by the end of September, they too decided to leave. Their departure left the hospital acutely short of medical and clerical staff, as well as attendants. To make matters worse, the supply of food, warm clothing, and medicines was disrupted. Muslim refugees began to pour in. And an outbreak of cholera killed a huge number of patients that winter. The year 1946 had seen a mortality rate of a little over 7 per cent. This surged to 17 per cent in 1947.

The next year was barely better. When Dr Lloyd Still – who had been at the helm for close to two years – left in the month of March, he was replaced by Dr Ahmad Shafi. However, posts of physicians continued to lie vacant. Refugees who had been engaged as attendants proved to be irregular and inefficient. Shortages persisted. Patients were reported to be 'badly nourished', even 'very nearly starving'. Most of them were in poor health. The mortality rate fell, but only marginally. Fourteen per cent of Lahore's patients died in 1948.

In December 1948, the governments of Pakistan and India finally agreed on what to do with mental patients whose relatives were on the other side. Such non-Muslim patients in Pakistan were supposed to be transferred to India. And Muslim patients in India were supposed to be transferred to Pakistan. But the patients would only be transferred after the two governments had sorted out their pending financial dues.

At this point, India had made a list of 240 patients who were to be sent to Pakistan. And Pakistan had made a list of 513 patients who were to be sent to India. Of these, 359 were then at the Lahore mental hospital, 106 were at the Hyderabad mental hospital in Sind, and 48 were in the mental barracks of Peshawar jail.

It was not clear how the two lists were drawn up. Millions of people had moved and thousands of people had died. Did the patients' relatives keep in touch with the respective hospitals? Did the authorities attempt to track them down? How many was it possible to trace? How many were never found? And what would happen to patients whose next of kin was not known?

In February 1949, a batch of 32 non-Muslim patients were transferred out of Lahore. After that, the process came to a halt. It stood still for almost two years.

~

Back in India, the government of East Punjab had decided to build its own mental hospital in Amritsar, a city just 50 kilometres from Lahore. It took quite a while to take this decision. In May 1948, it appointed Dr R.S. Sharma to get the project going. Dr Sharma had served as deputy superintendent at the Lahore mental hospital for several years, before taking over briefly as superintendent in 1939. He had, however, since retired from the provincial medical service. The site chosen for the hospital used to be a resettlement colony for certain nomadic communities, who were officially termed as 'criminal tribes'. A few of its buildings were usable, several had to be condemned.

Much of Amritsar was in shambles after the riots of 1947. The city was then in the process of being rebuilt. The scarcity of steel, cement, and labour slowed down repairs and construction of the hospital. And equipment, bedding, and clothing were hard to obtain. Though the work was yet to be finished, the hospital opened on 1 March 1949.

The Amritsar mental hospital was designed for about 400

patients. It admitted 103 local patients in its first year, including six who had recently been transferred from Lahore. A hundred beds were kept empty for others who were expected from across the border. When this would happen was not yet known.

Nineteen months went by.

In October 1950, *The Tribune* published the official list of Indian patients who had died at the Lahore mental hospital between 20 August 1947 and 23 July 1950. This list contained 143 names, along with their last known address. Several addresses were missing. The date of death was not reported, nor was its cause. Indian patients who may have died at Hyderabad and Peshawar did not figure in this list.

On 6 December 1950, the countries exchanged their mentally ill patients in a single simultaneous exercise. The two groups had first been assembled at the hospitals in Lahore and Amritsar respectively. By this time, the numbers had undergone a change. India transferred 233 patients to West Pakistan and received 450 patients in return. The 282 Indian patients who apparently belonged to East Punjab were admitted to the Amritsar mental hospital. And the 168 Indian patients who remained were sent to the mental hospital at Kanke.

The division of assets and liabilities between Pakistan and India was documented in great detail. But crucial details of the transfer of mentally ill patients have not yet been uncovered. How many patients had become foreigners after 15 August 1947? How was their fate decided? Were they treated differently from domestic patients? How many of them were discharged on an individual basis? And how many died before the two governments arranged for their transfer? None of this is known.

Why did the transfer of mentally ill patients take so long? After all, the two governments were able to evacuate over a quarter million of their citizens in a matter of months. Why then did it take them more than three years to reclaim a few hundred who were in mental hospitals? Each side had disputed the other's financial claims. Did that hold up the process of transfer? The two sides had agreed upon the simultaneous exchange of patients. Could that have taken excessive time to arrange? Or were the authorities simply busy with matters that they considered far more important? None of this is known.

What is, however, known is that the mental hospitals were public institutions, and their patients were in state care. The future of hundreds of patients became precarious when the subcontinent was divided. It was the responsibility of the two governments to protect the interests of these patients. Instead, they seem to have treated them no better than second-class citizens.

~

By 1951, things were falling into place at Lahore and at Amritsar. The two hospitals together took in four times the number of patients that had been admitted to Lahore in the year preceding partition. Unlike in the past, many of these were voluntary patients. In another new feature, both hospitals were treating a large number of outpatients as well. What had led to these changes? Were the hospitals now serving a bigger population than before? Did the process of partition trigger a rise in mental illness? Had it become more difficult for families to cope with their mentally ill on their own?

Partition had unleashed a wave of social turmoil, communal ferment, and personal tragedy that would devastate more generations than one. India's brand new government was clearly ill-equipped for this crisis. In the years to come, there would be a string of other crises. Some would be caused by human action, some would be inflicted by nature. Each such crisis could have an impact on the mental health of the people it affected. Would the state and society be better prepared by then?

> Frail and dressed in blue, Jagan Nath (87), who was shifted from Lahore's mental hospital to Amritsar in 1948 – a year after the Partition, gives an impression of a character of Urdu writer Saadat Hasan Manto's famous story – 'Toba Tek Singh'.
>
> The grey-haired Jagan Nath, who is still languishing in Dr Vidya Sagar Mental Hospital, here for the past 59 years does not know even the name of Pakistan … The record of Lahore's hospital, which too was sent to Amritsar, described the conduct of Jagan Nath as good. Jagan Nath was sentenced to one-year rigorous imprisonment in 1946 on charges of wandering.
>
> The Supreme Court order on the closure of cases against all those who had remained in judicial custody for more than the period of their sentences is unlikely to benefit Jagan Nath. Reason: his entire family is believed to have been killed in the communal frenzy of the Partition. Though he had completed his one year sentence in pre-Partition days, he still is living in his own world.[17]

---

[17] Varinder Walia, '59 Years Later, He Is Still Here', *The Tribune* (Chandigarh), 26 October 2007.

NINE

Bringing Out a Bill

This is what happened this morning. When I reached here, that gentleman was already occupying this seat. I questioned him. I felt doubtful whether he was a Member. I questioned him and asked him 'Are you a Member? Are you elected from some constituency?' He said 'Yes'. But he was very reserved. He would not answer. Ordinarily, when a new Member comes, rather he feels delighted to get introduced to other Members. But when I put two or three questions to him, he would hardly answer one. Then, I asked him whether he was a member of the Congress Party. He said, 'No'. Shri A. K. Gopalan was sitting behind me, and I asked him whether he was a member of his party. Shri A. K. Gopalan said, 'No'. Then, I asked him which party he belonged to, and he told me that he was an Independent. Then, I told him that this seat had already been allotted to the Leader of the Communist Party; I asked him why he was occupying this seat, and I told him that he should have gone to some other seat. He told me that the Speaker had put him there.

Meanwhile, you [Lok Sabha Speaker] entered in; if we had a couple of minutes more, perhaps, we would have discovered him. But then there was no time, and when you called on

Members to take oath, he at once came, and he was the first
to move out and take the oath.[18]

After the 1957 general election, parliament began its first session
in the month of May. Its members were sworn in over the next
few weeks, even as legislative business carried on. On 15 July
1957, a gentleman came forward to take his oath in the Lok
Sabha. He gave his name as Birendra Kumar Majumdar. Though
this name was not on the list, he insisted that he was a member.
He was sworn in, shook hands with the Speaker, and signed the
roll of members of parliament. At this point it was discovered
that he had indeed contested the election, but had lost. It also
appeared that he was 'mentally not sound'. The Speaker declared
that this was a 'serious affront to the dignity of the House'.
Prime Minister Jawaharlal Nehru suggested that members should
present their credentials in future, and this was then discussed for
a while.

A month later, the Speaker reported that the imposter had
been sent to a hospital and examined by a medical board. The
board decided that his was a case of 'schizo-phrenic reaction, a
type of insanity'. And the matter ended there.

No other person of unsound mind is known to have entered the
portals of parliament in those days. But some did appear in its
proceedings. In December 1950, one Nazir Khan had hoisted
a green flag on the Daulatabad Fort in Aurangabad. A member
asked if the flag was that of Pakistan, and if so, what action was
taken. A minister clarified that the flag was not that of Pakistan,
as it did not have a crescent. Besides, Nazir Khan had no political

---

[18] Sardar Hukam Singh's remarks, 'Question of Privilege', *Lok Sabha Debates*,
vol. III, no. 1 (15 July 1957): 3538–3539.

affiliations. He had apparently been dismissed from the police department on the grounds of being a 'lunatic'. Nazir Khan believed himself to be a saint who had renounced the world, and had merely hoisted the flag as an offering to the dargah. Under the circumstances, no action was taken against him. Nor was he offered any treatment. This explanation satisfied parliament.

In another instance, while speaking about arbitrary cases of preventive detention, a member cited the case of one Abdul Razak Khan. The charge against Khan was that he had reportedly said that he would raise an army in Manipur, and use it to occupy Pakistan and Calcutta. As a result, he was clapped in jail for three years without a trial. The member believed that Khan ought to have been sent to a 'lunatic asylum' instead of a jail. There was no discussion on the case.

The sudden 'mental collapse' of Professor Aleksandr F. Zelenovsky, a Russian national who worked at the Indian Statistical Institute in Calcutta, also came up in parliament. A medical examination showed that he was suffering from 'persecution mania' and an 'anxiety state with paranoid trends'. But there was speculation about the true facts of the case. Replying to a question from a member, Prime Minister Jawaharlal Nehru – who was also minister of external affairs – stated that he had no knowledge of Zelenovsky being harassed by Russians, or seeking Indian citizenship. He added that the professor had left for Moscow in January 1958. Curiously, a memorandum prepared by the Central Intelligence Agency in 1964 would claim that Zelenovsky had been whisked away by Soviet authorities because he had either attempted to defect, or was suspected of being on the verge of doing so. This, apparently, was how the Soviet Union often dealt with its dissidents.

Doubts also arose about the mental state of one G.D. Upadhyay, a central government employee. Once, while meeting with a superior officer, Upadhyay had been accompanied by a man toting a double-barrelled shotgun. Later, he had carried a gun himself when he went to see the same officer. So the officer in question had Upadhyay sent to the Agra mental hospital for observation. But Upadhyay's parents removed him from there before his medical report was ready. Was Upadhyay mentally ill? Nobody really knew. In the past, he had accused various officers of corruption. Had he been sent to an asylum for being a whistle-blower? The concerned minister did not think so, because some of Upadhyay's allegations were investigated and, in fact, found to be false. The subject was thereby closed.

During the 1950s and 1960s, parliament did not discuss mental illness very often. To the odd question posed, the concerned minister would usually reply that the subject was on the concurrent list. The central government's role was limited to legislation, research, and training. And while it did offer advice to state governments, the latter were free to take it or leave it. If asked about the incidence of mental illness, the minister simply repeated the conjectures that the Bhore committee had made back in 1946. As for mental hospitals in the country, there was little information other than their number. But the minister did take questions on the one at Ranchi, which the central government took over in 1954. And on the All India Institute of Mental Health, a centre for postgraduate training and research that was set up the following year at Bangalore.

A few pointed enquiries by members would also receive helpful replies. For instance, 18 per cent of defence personnel invalidated during World War II suffered from psychiatric disorders. By 1962, all large military hospitals had a psychiatry wing. Incidentally, all large general hospitals did not. In 1961, the centre had asked state governments for their views on setting up an all-India mental health service. Most states were against this. Mysore was the only one in favour of the proposal. Orissa preferred a central pool rather than a central service. So the proposal was dropped. A state of national emergency had been declared when the Indo-China war broke out in 1962. As several state governments were then short of funds, they cut back on mental health programmes. A 1967 study showed that 30 per cent of workers treated at the Rourkela Steel Plant were emotionally disturbed. Discussions in parliament revealed that the practice of keeping non-criminal patients in jail continued through the 1960s at several locations.

What did members of parliament think about mental illness in those days? Some clues are provided by their debates on sterilisation of the unfit.

In 1952, a private member's bill for the sterilisation of the unfit came up in the Lok Sabha. Its mover, S.V. Ramaswamy, said that it was a 'social tragedy to allow lepers, syphilitics, the insane, congenital idiots and the like to bring forth children'. His idea was not at all new. In USA, for instance, several states had enacted laws in the early 20th century for the forced sterilisation of the physically or mentally disabled, or of persons who were regarded as social deviants. Race, class, and gender, each had a place in the sterilisation programmes that were run in these states. California had apparently inspired the one that was launched in Nazi Germany in 1933. This had taken on a more macabre form during World War II, when hundreds of thousands – including young children – were selected for 'mercy death'. After the war, the horrors of these killings were revealed in the Nuremberg trials. And the scientific basis of eugenics was widely discredited. But forced sterilisation would remain legal in certain countries well into the 1970s.

Despite some support for Ramaswamy's bill, it died a quick

death. However, the subject surfaced again in the Rajya Sabha the very next year. Lilavati Munshi moved a resolution calling upon the government to enforce the sterilisation of adults suffering from incurable diseases or insanity. This, she argued, was necessary 'to save children and save the nation from being flooded with diseased people'. On her list of diseases were leprosy, tuberculosis, epilepsy, venereal diseases, drug addiction, and insanity. A fierce debate followed. Mona Hensman – whose husband had headed the Madras mental hospital for over a decade – was one of those who opposed the motion. But the most hard-hitting response came from health minister Rajkumari Amrit Kaur, who called it unscientific, unethical, and impractical. Refuting the notion that the listed illnesses were hereditary and incurable, she added that she would be 'very sorry to be a part and parcel of a government that indulges in violence of this nature'. Instead, she argued for more spending on health care. Lilavati Munshi had no choice but to withdraw her resolution.

Ten years passed before the subject resurfaced in the Rajya Sabha. Shakuntala Paranjpye, an eminent social worker, had introduced a private member's bill in 1964. This was finally taken up in parliament in 1969. Paranjpye pointed out that 'the normal healthy persons of the society are planning and limiting their families, while the sub-normal, the unhealthy and the diseased individuals go on procreating in an unrestricted manner'. She called for forced sterilisation 'for the social good, for public health, for the amelioration of our stock'. The principle, she suggested, was no different from that of compulsory vaccination. Once again, members swung into the debate. Some said that the bill was 'laudable' and offered their 'wholehearted' support. Others said that it was 'not at all necessary', 'worthless', even 'dangerous'. This time the government did not squash the bill at once. In fact, Dr S. Chandrasekhar, a demographer who was then the junior minister of health, agreed that it would be a good idea to seek public opinion. So the bill was circulated. While tuberculosis and mental illness experts had little to say, those dealing with leprosy opposed it roundly. Nevertheless, Paranjpye urged that the bill move to the next stage, that is, be referred to a select committee. She was keen that this should happen at once, as her term as a member of parliament was about to end.

Dr Chandrasekhar's response was tactful but firm. At the outset he stated that the very concept of compulsory sterilisation was 'rather repugnant to our attitudes and the cultural traditions of this country'. Leprosy, tuberculosis and numerous mental disorders were definitely curable. He would like to study the issue more deeply and see the experience of more advanced countries. And he promised to try to bring a 'more comprehensive and acceptable and constitutionally valid measure' before parliament 'at the appropriate time'. In conclusion, he requested Shakuntala Paranjpye to withdraw her bill. She refused. The question of taking the bill forward was put to a vote. That was the end of the bill.

~

Modern science saw mental disorder as a class of diseases that varied a great deal in form and degree. Though some could be severely disabling, others were decidedly less so. Their origin was pretty much a matter of speculation. But it was possible to classify them, to define methods of diagnosis, and to understand how they progressed over time. The treatment of mental disorder was led by two established fields of science – psychiatry and psychology. While the former sought to heal the human 'body', the latter dwelt on the human 'mind'. Psychiatrists and psychologists did not agree very often. But between them, they offered a range of therapies to those who were mentally ill. It was held that with suitable treatment and care, especially at an early stage, most illnesses could be managed, and many could be even be cured.

None of this figured in the way the law dealt with mental disorder in India.

Enacted in the year 1912, the Indian Lunacy Act placed mental illness on the same footing as mental retardation. Much of the law was about admission to a mental hospital. While it did allow these hospitals to take in voluntary patients, it concentrated on the involuntary ones. Those whose admission was not ordered by military or prison authorities had to come through a civil court. A special section of the law laid down how an affluent patient's property must be managed. But the law said nothing about the treatment or care of any patients at all.

In 1949, the Indian Psychiatric Society had called for a new mental health law in the country. A bill was then drafted by three of its members – Dr Robert Brockelesby Davis, Dr S.A. Hasib, and Dr Jyotirmay Roy. The society urged the government to take this draft forward. Support for a new law also came from Dr William Mayer-Gross, a leading psychiatrist who had been deputed by the World Health Organization to the Government of India. But the idea lay buried for a quarter of a century.

Despite two stints as health minister in the 1950s and 1960s, Dr Sushila Nayar had been unable to bring a new mental health bill before parliament. However, she did manage to do so as a private member, regretting the 'unconscionable' delay. When her bill came up for discussion in 1978, health minister Raj Narain announced that the government was actually ready with a bill of its own. The two then argued about whose bill was better. Eventually, Dr Nayar had to withdraw her bill, though she was 'not at all happy' about this. A few weeks later, the government introduced its bill, which was then handed over to a parliamentary committee. In a spirit of bonhomie, this committee was chaired by Dr Nayar.

The committee soon got to work. It studied 45 written memoranda, heard 17 witnesses, and visited various institutions in Agra, Bangalore, Calcutta, Delhi, Jammu, Lucknow, Madras, Ranchi, Srinagar, Tezpur, and Vizagapatam. It took about six months to present its report to parliament. But before this could be discussed, the government fell. In August 1979, the Lok Sabha was dissolved. Thus, the Mental Health Bill, 1978, lapsed.

Two years passed.

A revised bill was introduced in 1981 and entrusted to a new parliamentary committee in 1982. This committee received 37 memoranda, deposed 23 witnesses, and visited a number of places. But its progress was rather slow. By the time fresh elections were held two and half years later, it had yet to finish its task.

The bill was referred to a fresh committee in 1985. Wisely, this committee decided to pick up from where the previous one had left off. It therefore consulted just seven memoranda and five witnesses. Between them, the two committees had been to Agra, Benares, Calcutta, Delhi, Hyderabad, Madras, Nagpur, Panaji, Poona, Srinagar, Tezpur, Trivandrum, and Vizagapatam. Their visits covered mental hospitals, general hospitals, medical colleges, and prisons. They had met local officials and had even spoken with patients. The report of the committee was tabled within a year.

In the year 1987, parliament finally enacted a new law on mental health.

∼

After World War II, the western world began to think differently about mental health. And as accounts of abuse in mental hospitals came to light, these institutions fell into disrepute. Demands for reform became vocal, and medical ethics were keenly debated.

Meanwhile, psychiatry was galvanised by the discovery of mood stabilisers, antipsychotics, antidepressants, and anti-anxiety medications. These new drugs allowed patients with a range of disorders to spend far less time in a hospital. They also offered a range of treatments that could be administered to out-patients. However, the side effects of drugs, and the dangers of excessive medication were matters of public concern.

An anti-psychiatry movement took shape in the 1960s. Activists opposed the practice of treating patients against their will. They also held that patients had a right to be fully informed about what their treatment involved. Challenging the biomedical view of mental disorder, the movement stressed upon social, economic, and cultural contexts instead.

By the 1980s, many countries had chosen to bring in policies and programmes for treatment outside the mental hospital. Outpatient clinics and therapy centres sprang up, creating space for assorted mental health professionals. The population of mental hospitals declined. Some countries even did away with them altogether.

Things happened differently in India. When the country became independent in 1947, there was perceived to be a shortage of mental hospitals. Besides, the ones that existed were not evenly distributed. In 1951, there were 30 public and private facilities with a little over 10,000 beds. By 1986, the count stood at 45, most of which were run by government authorities. The number of beds had doubled. And annual admissions had shot up almost ten-fold. Unlike in the past, many of them offered outpatient services as well.

At the same time, a number of general hospitals and teaching hospitals had opened departments of psychiatry. This made it much simpler for people to seek treatment – as outpatients as well as inpatients. But the number of beds in psychiatric wards was no more than 10 to 15 per cent of those in mental hospitals. As far as inpatient care was concerned, mental hospitals were there to stay. The public did not question the way these hospitals were being run.

Psychiatry had taken an early lead over clinical psychology. As of 1985, there were about a thousand qualified psychiatrists in India, as against possibly four to five hundred clinical psychologists. Psychotropic drugs and electroconvulsive treatment were liberally prescribed for all sorts of mental illnesses. The public did not question the way psychiatry was being practiced. Nor did it demand alternative forms of therapy.

The Indian Mental Health Act of 1987 was supposed to bring in 'the latest concepts and knowledge' in the field. It called for the central government and for every state government to set up an authority to advise it on all matters relating to mental health. These bodies were also supposed to regulate institutions – public and private – that provided mental health services. Hospitals, nursing homes, convalescent homes, halfway houses, and other facilities – whether general or specialised – figured on this list. For the very first time, mental health was set to become visible in public policy and practice.

Other than that, the law devoted itself solely to mental hospitals and mental nursing homes. Each had to be headed by a psychiatrist. And each had to treat outpatients as well as in-patients. Both of these conditions had been unthinkable in the early 20th century.

Like the colonial law that it replaced, the new one was mostly about admission and discharge. There were, however, vital differences. Unlike in the past, a patient could now be admitted for short-term treatment without a court order. This would come as a big relief to many. The powers of a magistrate were clipped some more. He no longer had the discretion to decide where to send a patient for observation. Now that 'proper medical custody' was specified, jail was ruled out as a destination. Once a magistrate decided that a patient needed to be admitted to a mental hospital or nursing home, there might be some delay in carrying this out. In the old days, the patient could end up waiting indefinitely in jail. Under the new law, a magistrate had to choose an 'appropriate' place where a patient could stay temporarily. He had to record his reasons for this decision. And he had to specify the duration of stay, which could not exceed a period of thirty days.

In the new scheme of things, doctors had a bigger role in the admission and discharge of patients. But the law sidestepped some difficult questions. Did the patient have any say in his admission and treatment? What kinds of therapies were allowed? And what were the standards for treatment and care to be followed?

A separate chapter of the new law dealt exclusively with 'human rights'. It was strangely brief. To begin with, no patient was to be subjected to indignity or cruelty. But the law did not explain either term. Second, no patient was to be used as a research subject without his consent. But the law did not state how to verify such consent. If a patient was not competent to make this decision, his guardian could do so on his behalf. But the law did not say how competence was to be judged. Either way, doctors could simply go ahead with any research that they thought would help a patient. Third, a patient was free to write and to receive letters. But the law allowed these to be intercepted, detained, or destroyed if they were harmful for the patient. Or if they were vexatious or defamatory to the institution. Clearly, none of these three 'human rights' were absolute. And together they fell way short of what every patient deserved.

Thanks to a series of procedural hiccups, the Mental Health Act of 1987 only came into force in the year 1993. With that, the Indian Lunacy Act of 1912 was finally repealed. The new law was certainly without some of the flaws of the old. But it did have flaws of its own. The most glaring one was that it failed to protect the rights of the mentally ill – whether inside mental health institutions or outside them.

~

Parliament reflected all shades of opinion that were to be found in society at large. Was mental illness a result of supernatural forces? Planetary influences? Bad genes? Diseased brains? Did it make a person dangerous? Irrational? Incompetent? Useless? A burden on society? Who was responsible for persons who were mentally ill? And how should this responsibility be handled? Each question opened up many more.

There were, of course, plenty of enlightened answers. But there was also ignorance, prejudice, and apathy. Perhaps this explains why it took so long to enact a new law. It might also explain why this law would not sweep in the winds of change.

Mental illness seems to have very close connection with lunar position. Mr. Vice-Chairman, you know the word 'lunatic' came out of 'lunar' which means the moon. It is a well-known observation that mentally ill persons rave mad during the time when it is new moon day or the full moon day. Scientists both from India and Australia have established recently a very close connection between the lunar position and mental illness. This means that in our mental hospitals, the doctors should be careful on those days and see that nothing untoward should happen. This is an important observation which I would like to make because the mental hospitals should be particularly alert on those days. I do not know but there is a predication that children born on new moon and full moon days, that is, when the moon is at its zenith or nadir – the opposite point – are said to have tendencies to have mental illnesses.[19]

[19] Prof. B. Ramachandran Rao's remarks, 'The Mental Health Bill, 1981', *Rajya Sabha Official Debates, Part 2 – Other than Question and Answer* (25 November 1986): 266, http://rsdebate.nic.in/handle/123456789/321321.

TEN

Inside Stories

Ward boys showed this correspondent wooden planks that they had put up on crumbling doors and windows. 'If a patient escapes or jumps to his death, we are the ones who will be punished. And, therefore, we have no alternative but to collect money ourselves and somehow do the work,' said one of them. This correspondent also saw a window in Block number three where broken cots had been placed to block a gaping window in a pathetic attempt to prevent accidents. Most of the ward boys were found sitting on gunny bags on the floor.

What was even more horrifying was to find the patients huddled on the bare floor, most of them scratching their lice-infested bodies. Some of them, in sheer desperation, had taken off their shirts. Some of them had not bathed for weeks. All of them were wearing the same set of clothes given to them three weeks ago. None of the wards visited by this correspondent had any bathroom. During the monsoon, the only bath the inmates have is when they are soaked in the rain.

The few cots in the wards were full of bugs. A ward boy lifted a cot and then let it fall with a thud. Bugs virtually rained on the floor.

On the first floor of the Blocks, big, dirty drums were kept to store drinking water fetched from the ground floor. The toilets were filthy.

This correspondent spent an hour-and-a-half visiting four wards but he did not come across a single nursing staff or doctor. The attendants said nurses visit the wards for an hour in the morning and for another hour in the afternoon while the doctors rarely venture out of their chambers.[20]

Clamping down on political unrest in the country, Prime Minister Indira Gandhi got the President of India to proclaim a state of national emergency in June 1975. What followed was the suspension of democracy and rule by decree. Dissent was quelled by the detention of opposition leaders. Citizens' civil liberties were curbed. And the press was muzzled through censorship, controls, and intimidation. The emergency was finally lifted in March 1977 and general elections were held. A bunch of opposition parties had come together to form the Janata Party. Together with its allies, it won 298 seats against the Congress score of 153. For the first time in three decades, the Congress was voted out of power at the centre. Soon after, it would also lose in a number of states where it had held office.

The Janata government undid the controversial measures of the past two years, and probed the excesses of the outgoing regime. It, however, did not survive for very long. Elections took place in 1980. And this time the Congress triumphed. With 351 members in the lower house of parliament, it dominated the treasury benches once again.

The dramatic events of the late 1970s had spurred a great deal of public interest in current affairs. At the same time, new

---

[20] Uttam Sengupta, 'The Asylum from which the Inmates Escaped', *The Telegraph*, 8 September 1984.

technologies for communication and for printing were on offer. And the growth of corporate advertising came as a big boost to the media industry. The number of daily newspapers and their circulation figures almost doubled over the decade – a trend that would continue in the 1980s. An assortment of magazines and other periodicals came to be launched. Bright young men and women were drawn to journalism in a big way. And conventional coverage began to make more space for investigative reports that scrutinised political moves, questioned government action and inaction, and confronted social wrongs.

The mentally ill did not make it to the national news very often. When they did, it was for all the wrong reasons.

Before independence, the Indian Mental Hospital, Kanke, was regarded as a modern institution, a fine example for others to follow. It is not clear when exactly this stopped being true. But by the early 1980s, there were plenty of reasons for it to be in the news.

In June 1982, *India Today* carried an article on the hospital, which by then was called the Ranchi Mansik Arogyashala. The grim account by Chaitanya Kalbag described it as 'crawling with decay and despair'. Everything assailed the senses, from the sight of men and women living in conditions 'that make the word squalid sound respectable', to the smell of 'uncared-for bodies' that inhabited 'shockingly maintained' wards. Many patients had to 'rot for years' after being certified as sane, because their relatives would not take them back. Women were more likely than men to be abandoned in this fashion.

The accompanying photographs by Raghu Rai left little to the imagination. One was of newly arrived patients tied to iron bed-frames, unclothed. Dogs and patients were seen eating from the same plates in the women's section. A scene from the kitchen showed chapatis being rolled out on a filthy floor. And in another, a patient was being held down by four men, while a fifth held out a primitive pincer-like contraption in the 'shock shop'.

Understaffed and underfunded, the hospital authorities were apparently trying to make the best of an impossible situation. Yet the medical superintendent had candidly admitted that his patients were worse off than the inmates of a concentration camp.

Two years later, the hospital was in the news again. On 4 September 1984, the lower staff had gone on strike to protest a pay cut. This left the patients unfed as well as unguarded. The next morning, 276 of them wandered out of the hospital gates. The strike was called off the following day, and order was restored. But before that had happened, a young reporter named Uttam Sengupta managed to sneak inside with a photographer. *The Telegraph* carried the story on the 8th of September, and tracked it over the coming weeks. Digging into the past, the paper printed charges of negligence, malpractice, and corruption that the Bihar government had allegedly chosen to ignore.

A week after the 'escape', 188 patients had been 'captured', while 88 remained 'at large'. But the bigger story was the eyewitness account of 'disgraceful living conditions' at the hospital. A few wards on the ground floor were 'showpieces' for the benefit of visiting dignitaries. Unlike these, the wards on the first floor were usually kept locked. They were badly maintained, poorly ventilated, and ill-lit. And they had neither cots nor mattresses. Sengupta also learnt that the hospital did not have a morgue. Corpses were seen 'carelessly dumped' in a corner of a ward. The fate of the dead, he pointed out, was hardly surprising when one witnessed the treatment meted out to the living.

∼

A sprinkling of disturbing articles had appeared in the press during the 1980s and 1990s. Kanke was not the only mental hospital to be singled out. The reportage included stories from Agra, Ahmedabad, Amritsar, Bangalore, Calicut, Gwalior, Nagpur, Ranchi, Ratnagiri, Thane, and Yeravda.

Were all mental hospitals in the same situation? And did all patients get a raw deal? That was not the case. The stories of those who were treated well, whose condition improved, and who returned to their home would remain untold.

In October 1981, Sreedhar Pillai reported that two male attendants at the Calicut mental hospital allegedly got drunk and climbed the outer wall of the women's ward. One of them then unlocked the heavy iron door of a cell, and assaulted its inmate – 26-year-old Premaja. The other attendant happened to drop the bunch of keys as he tried to enter the next cell. The noise woke up its two inmates. They raised an alarm and the culprits fled.

After keeping quiet for the next three days, Premaja confided in the head nurse. The hospital, however, hushed things up. When a group of its employees leaked the story, the police registered a case. There was a public uproar, protests were held outside the hospital, and local organisations came forward to champion Premaja's cause. Her father, a retired school teacher, wrote to the prime minister and the chief minister, demanding action against the criminal negligence of the authorities. According to him, his daughter suffered from depressive psychosis. Except for the occasional violent outburst, she was well-behaved. She had been in the hospital for the past 12 years.

It was not unheard of for a magistrate to send a mentally ill person to jail until he could be admitted to a mental hospital. This was the practice in Madhya Pradesh, as also in various other states. In June 1982, Sreekant Khandekar found that there were 34 such 'non-criminal lunatics' at Gwalior's central jail. The jail authorities said that the Gwalior mental hospital would not take them. And the hospital authorities said that the jail had not sent them over. As a result, these patients remained in jail. At least four of them had been waiting there for more than eight years.

While they waited, these men were living in a long, narrow hall, which they shared with mentally ill convicts and undertrials. Raised cement slabs served as beds for the inmates. A psychiatrist from the Gwalior mental hospital visited the jail, but these visits were neither frequent nor regular. Patients could be taken to the mental hospital for consultation, as it was just 200 yards away from the jail. But, like all prisoners, they could only be moved under police escort. And it was not always possible to arrange for this facility.

In a complaint to the Bombay High Court in July 1988, H.A. Shukri alleged that his mother had died of negligence at Yeravda. The court then appointed a commission to look into all four mental hospitals in Maharashtra. The commissioner's report led the court to observe that patients in these hospitals were 'treated like animals'. It ordered the state government to carry out several improvements. Six months later, *The Times of India* reported that not much had changed.

Yeravda's buildings were still dilapidated, with leaking ceilings, torn netting, broken doors, ripped electrical fittings, damaged compound walls, and a 'terrible shortage of water and toilets'. A journalist who had been recently admitted for de-addiction claimed that the attendants were cruel to patients. They would, for instance, take an 'excited' patient to the 'oonch ward', where criminal patients were locked up. One such patient had returned with a broken leg. The journalist had also seen other patients brought back battered and bleeding to the infirmary. At times, an attendant would beat up a patient just 'for the fun of it'. During Holi celebrations that year, drunk attendants had tied two patients to a tree and whipped them with leather belts. On another occasion, a patient with high fever was given a hot bath and left to dry in the sun, after which he developed complications and died.

Most of the patients at the overcrowded Nagpur hospital were chronic cases. One of them had been there since 1929. The *Times of India* correspondent came across three alcoholics 'bunched together' with 60 epileptic patients. Among them was a child. The isolation cells at Nagpur were 8'x6' cages with rusty iron grills. They were smaller than enclosures for animals in a zoo.

Like Nagpur, Thane too was overcrowded. The hospital had only 300 beds for its 1,756 patients. These beds were reserved for those who had recovered. No bedding was given to any patient, not even in winter. After meals, patients drank water, tea, or milk from their thali, as neither glasses nor mugs were provided. Most of them bathed in the open.

The smallest of the four mental hospitals, Ratnagiri was also overcrowded. It was short of trained staff, and faced delays in medical supplies. In very many cases, relatives did not take back patients who had recovered.

Under the law, a person cannot be tried for a crime unless he is of sound mind. So when a mentally ill person is charged with an offence, his trial may have to be postponed till he is declared capable of defending himself in court. All this while, he is supposed to be treated for his condition – in jail or at a mental hospital. Also, his mental state is supposed to be periodically assessed. Under the law, a mentally ill undertrial may remain in jail or a mental hospital indefinitely.

In May 1992, Ramesh Vinayak reported that there were 22 undertrials at the Amritsar mental hospital. Some had been accused of murder. Others were charged with trivial crimes. Gattu, for instance, had been arrested for stealing cigarettes 15 years ago. And Bawa Singh was picked up for trespassing at the age of 26. He was now 53. If tried, and if convicted, these persons would have been handed a jail sentence that was far shorter than the time they had spent at the hospital. But most of them were unlikely to ever appear in court.

One such person was Raksha Devi, who had been accused of killing her husband ten years ago. Her daughter, Meenu, was born at the Amritsar mental hospital. Bright and quick-witted, the child lived with her mother in a hospital ward.

Writing for the *Indian Express* in June 1994, Siraj Qureshi revealed that a number of patients at the Agra mental hospital were actually 'quite normal'. But their relatives were not willing to take them home. This was not particularly surprising, for they had been 'packed off' to the hospital for 'piquant reasons' that had nothing to do with their state of mind. According to Qureshi, the hospital was using electroconvulsive therapy as 'first aid', and fellow-patients were made to assist in the procedure. A female patient had a fractured hand from being beaten by an attendant. And hooligans had entered the women's ward through the broken boundary wall. Qureshi's article was based on an official inquiry by assistant district magistrate Hardev Singh, who had been tipped off about a racket in fake medical certificates.

Qureshi's article was followed by three more. Usha Rai, who made a trip to the hospital, saw for herself its decrepit buildings, leaking roofs, and broken walls. Many patients in the male wards were stark naked, some lay in their own faeces and urine. Attendants who wished to 'play hookey' gathered patients into one ward and locked them in. There would be two or three persons to a bed, while others were on the floor. Several of the iron beds had no mattress. Women were not provided sanitary napkins when they menstruated. Instead, they were simply locked in a cell for a few days. Some patients who were infested with lice had gouged out holes in their scalp. The procedure for electroconvulsive therapy reminded Rai of an abbatoir. After a cloth bag was placed over the patients' heads, they would be 'dragged off kicking and screaming like goats for slaughter'. And while the shock was being administered, they were held down by 'other terrified patients'.

Thanks to Hardev Singh's inquiry, a committee of doctors at the hospital reviewed a large number of cases, and declared that 180 patients were mentally sound. Around 80 of them were quickly released. The rest were held back for a second opinion. In the meantime, Hardev Singh was transferred.

Usha Rai had raised a pertinent point at the time – 'If a government which has come to power on the votes of the marginalised, cannot run efficiently one mental hospital with a little over 400 patients, can it run a whole state?'

India Today published a piece by Farzand Ahmed and Avirook Sen in September 1996. The photo-feature was about persons who had been abandoned by their relatives at one mental hospital or another.

Born in a poor farming family in Karnataka, Narsamma had been married at the age of five. After a miscarriage at 16, she slid into manic depression. Deserted by her husband, she went to live with her brothers for a while, before wandering off on her own. In 1977 she was brought to NIMHANS – the National Institute of Mental Health and Neurosciences – in Bangalore. Within a few months, she became stable. Her brothers were contacted and they took her home. But she did not receive either the medicine or the compassion that would keep her well. Each time she relapsed, she was brought back to the hospital. The third such instance was in 1980. This time, an attendant from NIMHANS took Narsamma home when she improved. The two women were literally chased away from there. Later that year it was found that Narsamma's relatives had moved without leaving a forwarding address. By 1982, the hospital gave up trying to reach them. Sixteen years after she should have been discharged, Narsamma was still at the hospital. Now 60 years old, the only medicines she needed were those to control her blood pressure.

Rajkumari was diagnosed with schizophrenia when she was 26. Treated at the Ahmedabad mental hospital in 1990, she improved dramatically in just three months. Having been put on medication, she was soon fit for discharge. Rajkumari was an orphan, and her uncle refused to be her guardian. So she was sent to a home for destitute women. But she did not stay there for long. Some of the women would throw stones at her and taunt her as insane. She relapsed, and was back at the hospital in a month and a half. Ten months later, the Mahila Vikas Griha was persuaded to take her in once again. This time she only lasted two days. The abuse was too much for her. She was out of control, crying to be taken back to the hospital. As its attempts to rehabilitate her had failed, the hospital decided to let her stay on. Unlike in the outside world, she would face no stigma there. Upon being asked what she missed most, she jokingly replied, 'Let me think … samosas. Yes, that's about the only good thing there is outside.'

In 1996, there were around 40 patients at the Ranchi Mansik Arogyashala who were considered stable. One of them was Pranab Mukhopadhyay. Unlike Narsamma and Rajkumari, he was from a well-to-do family. A former employee at the Calcutta Municipal Corporation, he was diagnosed as schizophrenic in 1970. Four years later, the doctors decided that he could go home. But his relatives did not show up to collect him. Nor did they come to visit. Apparently his mother had forbidden them to do so. When she passed away in 1988, his younger brother finally came to see him. After years of total silence, this was the first time that Pranab met a member of his family. But that did not mean that he could go home. 'I don't exist anymore for my relatives and friends,' he told the reporter, 'so where do I go if I leave here?' By this time he was working as a typist-cum-stenographer at the hospital. Every now and then he was asked to type out a letter of discharge for a patient. That patient would never be him.

After spending a year at the Agra mental hospital, Shail Batra was certified as symptom-free in 1983. But her husband – an engineer with the public works department – refused to take her home. While Shail remained at the hospital, her husband and daughter visited her once a year. In 1994, the hospital started a drive to discharge patients who had been there for a long time. When it tried to persuade Shail's husband to take her home, he simply stopped visiting his wife. Shail did not give up. Every fortnight, she would submit an application to the hospital authorities, asking them to contact her husband. 'I've written to him as well,' she said, 'but I don't think the letters have reached him.'

Harpreet Kaur was brought to the Agra mental hospital by her husband, who complained that she was violent and unmanageable. The doctors did not think that Harpreet was mentally ill, but they decided to keep her under observation. At the end of this period, they found no reason to admit her, and asked her husband to take her home. He refused. It turned out that he wanted his wife out of the way as he was living with another woman.

Before he fell ill, Chiman Patel worked in his brother's factory. He improved after being treated at the Ahmedabad mental hospital. In an experiment to encourage patients to learn to live a somewhat independent life, five patients were moved out of their ward to an empty staff quarter on the campus. One of them was Chiman. Chiman worked at a handloom unit at the hospital, and even had a light job in the city for a while. Then 28 years old, he had announced, '… I am in control now, I can go back.' The doctors did not tell him that on more than one occasion, his brother had asked them if there was 'any way of putting him to sleep'.

When he was 30 years old, Ashok Kumar Shukla was admitted to the Agra mental hospital in a manic state. That was in 1981. The doctors found him fit for discharge after some months. Yet, 15 years later, he was still there. His father, a senior government officer, clearly did not want him back. Each time the hospital prepared to discharge him, it received a letter from a random government department – agriculture, housing, even the Muslim Wakf Board – stating that Ashok had a serious illness and must be treated properly. The hospital got the message. Unaware of this correspondence, Ashok continued to believe that his father would have a change of heart. All this while, he had received only one letter from home. His younger sister had written to him 12 years ago, and he had memorised her words. 'She wrote that she missed me very much,' he recalled, 'and wanted me to come home. And that I should brush my teeth, wear clean clothes and bathe regularly.'

~

Among various articles that appeared in the press, 'Hell of a Cure' stands out as a rare personal account. Written by Anjana Mishra, it was carried by *Manushi* in the year 2000. Anjana had spent nine months and ten days at one of the better mental hospitals in the country – the Central Institute of Psychiatry, Ranchi. For her, this was a time of 'soul-destroying monotony … [that] spelt utter helplessness and despair'.

Anjana wrote of wards tightly packed with cots, of filthy toilets that had no water, of bathing in verandahs, of the use of ropes to tie women who were considered violent. She also described in great detail the dining hall with dirty tables, where some patients ate on the floor with dogs, and used plates were merely dipped in a drum of water to clean them. Life in the hospital was ruled by the attending ayahs. Patients were forced to carry out chores, which included washing the soiled clothes of others who were sick. Those who refused to obey got the 'cold water treatment' – being dunked in a tub of cold, dirty water. Nobody dared complain.

A victim of an abusive marriage, Anjana had been brought to Ranchi in July 1996 by her husband, an Indian Forest Service officer. A week later, she was declared 'normal'. Though the hospital wrote to her husband several times, he did not care to respond. Back in Orissa, her father appealed to the State Human Rights Protection Cell for help. An inspector arrived in Ranchi to look into her case and recommended that she be released. But this did not happen. Finally, her father got in touch with Utkal Mahila Samiti, a leading women's organisation. This time the State Human Rights Protection Cell took charge of the situation.

Anjana Mishra was rescued in April 1997. As she left the hospital, her fellow inmates pleaded with her to get them freed too.

> Now that I am back in the 'saner' world, my painful memories take me back frequently to the heartrending scenes of young mothers, separated from their tender infants, clinging and

singing lullabies to bundles of clothing. One then realizes that real life is not much different from reel life, and that real life is often very realistically portrayed in reel life.

Yet, amidst all that gloom, agony and despair, with inmates bereft of any hope but still yearning for freedom, in the face of death and degradation, I witnessed rare glimpses of humanity.

Having lived all these months with so-called 'abnormal and insane' people, I realised how mistaken our belief is and how false our illusions are about 'sanity'. The peacefulness inside me is in stark contrast to the violent and dangerous world outside. These so-called 'insane people' are actually simple, innocent and harmless souls, blessed with extraordinary sensitivity and totally bereft of the complexities of human nature, such as jealousy and hatred. Except on rare occasions, I never saw physical fights between the patients in CIP. Instead, I saw a human bond between them of which I too became a part. That bond survives even today.[21]

---

[21] Anjana Mishra, 'First Person – Hell of a Cure', *Manushi*, no. 120 (September–October 2000): 16.

ELEVEN

Breaking the Law

Shri Dasaratha Deb: Will the Minister of Health and Family Planning be pleased to state:

(a) whether Government are aware that a number of insane persons are kept in the different Jails of India, particularly in Bihar[,] where there are no qualified doctors for treating mental diseases;

(b) if so, why the insane or lunatic persons are kept for years in such Jails; and

(c) the reasons for not keeping them in mental hospitals or lunatic asylums where there are specialists in mental diseases?[22]

It was by no means a secret that an 'insane person' could wind up in jail without being charged of any crime whatsoever. This had, in fact, been going on for years. But, as Dr Sushila Nayar told members of parliament, it was only happening in some states, not all. At times, a person had to be kept under medical observation – for a short while – to check whether he was 'really insane'. For this purpose, he could be sent to a jail. If found

---

[22] Question asked by Dasaratha Deb, 'Lunatic Asylums', *Lok Sabha Debates*, vol. LI, no. 13 (3 March 1966): 3571.

'really insane', he would then be transferred to a mental hospital. But some hospitals had a long waiting list. In such a situation, his stay in jail had to be extended. The minister clarified that 'almost all' these jails offered treatment by qualified doctors. She also announced that the Indian Lunacy Act would be amended, so that state governments were obliged to provide 'suitable places' where a person's mental condition could be assessed.

While that summed up the official position in the year 1966, things were quite different in the early 1980s.

In the year 1981, there were 2077 'non-criminal lunatics' in various jails across the country. These jails were located in 13 of the 22 states, and in three of the nine union territories. West Bengal was in the lead with 1,301 patients, 380 of whom were women. With 404 patients, including 105 women, Assam came in second. Delhi – the national capital – was harbouring 22 patients in Tihar jail at the time. Many 'non-criminal lunatics' had been forced to live in inhuman conditions for years. They did not, in fact, receive proper treatment and care. And the Indian Lunacy Act was yet to be amended.

~

Little was heard on the subject till a 55-year-old convict died at Calcutta's Dum Dum jail on 8 January 1983. Claiming that his death was caused by lack of food and medical attention, the inmates went on hunger strike. That night, two 'non-criminal lunatics' also died. One was 25, and the other 27. They had been at Dum Dum for four and three years respectively. The inmates intensified their stir, refused to part with the three bodies, and demanded a meeting with the minister in charge of West Bengal's jails. The minister arrived on the morning of the 10th, and agreed to look into the prisoners' complaints. After that, the strike was called off. All this was covered in the press.

That same day, Rajesh Khaitan, an advocate who was a member of the legislative assembly, had petitioned the Calcutta High Court to intervene. Justice P.C. Barooah ordered the chief reporters of two leading dailies, *The Statesman* and *The Telegraph*, to visit the jail and inquire into its living conditions. It also asked the government of West Bengal for its initial response.

On the 25th of January, the two journalists handed in their reports. Apparently, the one by Sujoy Sengupta of *The Statesman* was 'mellower' than the one by Tarun Ganguly of *The Telegraph*. The judge allowed both reports to be published. But he held back certain observations on 'non-criminal lunatics' in Ganguly's report. Ganguly had also submitted various photographs and tape recordings of interviews. These were not to be published until the court so ordered.

What did Ganguly's report say? It basically said that the conditions at Dum Dum were dreadful. And that children – most of whom were 'mentally retarded' – and 'non-criminal lunatics' got the worst treatment.

Under the law, a 'non-criminal lunatic' could not be held in jail for more than 30 days. This law was being routinely broken. Anil Khasnobis, for instance, had arrived in 1953 at the age of 35. Amulya Chaudhury and Harimohan Dey had put in 26 and 23 years respectively. Cases such as theirs had not been reviewed since November 1967.

'Non-criminal lunatics' dressed in 'bug-infested rags' huddled together in crowded wards 'adorned with bugs lining the walls'. They were looked after by 'convict assistants', most of whom were lifers. When a usually calm 'lunatic' became violent, he was handcuffed and chained to a window till he became 'normal'. Habitually violent 'lunatics' were kept in a separate section. Ganguly saw about 50 of them, naked, patiently waiting for their meal. An official said that their clothes had gone for washing. A 'convict assistant' told Ganguly that they were not given any clothes, nor were they given any medicines.

There were, on an average, 703 'non-criminal lunatics' at Dum Dum. Yet the jail did not have a psychiatrist. The chief medical officer of the city's jails 'freely admitted' that only tranquilisers were ever prescribed. He was, however, not sure whether either food or medicine were reaching the 'lunatics' at all. A senior jail official 'casually admitted' that 10 to 12 of them died every winter.

Five days after reading the two reports, Justice Barooah paid a surprise visit to the jail. As he went around the premises and took photographs, he noticed certain improvements. Some 'non-criminal lunatics' were wearing brand new clothes. Some of the sick had been given 'factory fresh' red blankets. Walls once stained with the blood of squashed insects had been sand-papered. Yet, he found the conditions 'most shocking'.

The case came up in court on the 11th of February. Counsels for the jail authorities and the state government gave their side of the story. They also urged Justice Barooah to ignore Ganguly's report.

So far, *The Telegraph* had not published any of the photographs taken by Tapan Das, who had accompanied Ganguly to the jail. But *Sunday* magazine – a sister concern – came out with a selection of photographs on the 13th of February. *The Telegraph* followed suit four days later. As a result, the two periodicals were charged with contempt of court.

M.J. Akbar, who happened to be the editor of both, defended his decision – in print as well as in court. He said that until the photographs came in, he had no idea how bad things were at the jail. As a journalist, he believed it was his duty to expose the 'damning proof' of this 'horror' to as many readers as he could. The photographs were 'a million times more damaging' because they revealed the 'harsh truth' as no words could. Akbar stated that he did not intend any disrespect to the court by publishing them without its permission.

What did these photographs show? They showed a decrepit kitchen, a crumbling roof, a pile of rotting sack-cloth, a tattered blanket. They showed children, some naked, some physically disabled, some 'mentally retarded'. They showed prisoners, some emaciated, eating substandard food in dirty and broken utensils. They showed the walls of the 'lunatic block' smeared with the remains of dead insects. And they showed 'lunatics' lined up for food, most of them without any clothes.

The photographs were indeed horrifying. To Justice Barooah, they 'conclusively' established that the prisoners – 'non-criminal lunatics' in particular – were deprived of basic human rights. On the 24th of February he ruled, among other things, that all 'non-criminal lunatics' should be transferred to mental hospitals. If this was not possible, immediate steps should be taken to keep them in 'more congenial and healthy' surroundings. And till then, they should be looked after by paramedical staff, rather than by convicts.

In view of the 'extraordinary facts and circumstances' of the case, the charges against M.J. Akbar were later dropped. Although Akbar had indeed violated a court order, this did not amount to disrespect of the court. Nor did it impede the course of justice. Justice Barooah simply reprimanded Akbar and hoped that he would be 'more careful' in future. He also commended him for acting in the wider public interest.

The press had a long history as a defender of public interest. On the other hand, public interest litigation was of rather recent origin. Well into the 1970s, only an affected party could approach a court. But since then, the Supreme Court had taken up a series of cases that were filed by others on behalf of an affected party. High Courts would follow its lead. For those who were unable to go to court themselves, this was a rare chance to be heard. By the early 1980s, public interest litigation had caught on as a way for public-spirited citizens to seek judicial review of the actions – or inaction – of public authorities.

In January 1989, Sheela Barse wrote a letter to the Supreme Court, saying that 'non-criminal lunatics' had been illegally jailed in West Bengal. This was not her first foray into public affairs. As a freelance journalist, Barse had interviewed several women in Bombay Central Jail. In 1982, she petitioned the Supreme Court on their behalf. Two years later, she went to the Bombay High Court with a complaint against an observation home for children. Not satisfied with its ruling, she filed an appeal in the Supreme Court. In 1985, she turned to the Supreme Court once again on the issue of child prisoners in the country. And in 1986, she was invited to serve on a national expert committee that looked at how prisons and other institutions dealt with women in their custody. Her travels for this purpose may well have introduced Barse to 'non-criminal lunatics' in West Bengal's jails.

The Supreme Court asked the West Bengal government to explain itself, which it did. But the court was not satisfied. In June 1992, it appointed a two-member commission to look into a host of issues. One member was Professor Srinivasa Murthy, then head of the psychiatry department at the National Institute of Mental Health and Neurosciences, Bangalore. The other was

 Daman Singh

Dr Amita Dhanda, an assistant professor at the Indian Law Institute in Delhi. Murthy and Dhanda visited jails, mental hospitals, and social organisations and spoke with officials, magistrates, doctors, social workers, and patients. In January 1993, they submitted a two-volume report aptly titled *Unlock the Padlock: Mental Health Care in West Bengal.*

West Bengal held most 'non-criminal lunatics' in its five central jails. The commissioners learnt that Dum Dum central jail was short of beds, mattresses, fans, toilets, and bathrooms. They also found the food and clothing unsatisfactory. About a third of the patients were locked up in cells as they were considered 'disturbed'. Presidency jail was short of beds, mattresses, and toilets too. It confined some of its 'disturbed' women in 6'x6' cages. Alipore, Berhampore, and Midnapore jails did not have any beds. Whereas a jail might have certain facilities for recreation and rehabilitation of prisoners, these were denied to those who were mentally ill.

Presidency and Dum Dum were dubbed as specialised centres for mental patients. But neither had a psychiatrist, or any other mental health professional. A visiting psychiatrist came over to see patients from time to time. It could be weeks, even months, before he saw a new admission. Presidency kept an erratic medical record of each patient. Dum Dum, on the other hand, relied solely on verbal prescriptions. At both places, drugs were doled out to patients by convicts. Things at the other jails were similar, if not worse.

How did so many 'non-criminal lunatics' find their way to West Bengal's jails?

The law said that when somebody who seemed to be mentally ill was picked up by the police, he had to be brought before a magistrate. The magistrate was then supposed to examine the person. If he believed that there were grounds for pursuing the case, he would have to get him assessed by a medical officer. He could detain the person for medical observation for up to 10 days. Later, he could extend this period, but only up to 10 days at a time. And nobody could be held for more than 30 days in all. Once a medical officer had certified that a person was indeed mentally ill, the case was to go back to the magistrate. At this point, the magistrate could order the person to be admitted to a mental hospital within a month. Or, he could set him free.

The Indian Lunacy Act did not decide what places were suitable for medical observation. Each state government decided this for itself. In West Bengal, the list covered mental hospitals, general hospitals, and dispensaries. It also included jails, sub-jails, and lock-ups. It was, therefore, perfectly legal to send a person to jail for observation – for no more than 30 days.

But Murthy and Dhanda discovered that the law was being violated in all sorts of ways. To begin with, a person was not necessarily examined by a magistrate. Nor was a medical opinion necessarily called for. Instead, he was promptly sent to jail for 10 days or more. When this time was up, he was brought before the magistrate, with or without a medical report. His detention was then extended, with or without a time limit. In effect, a 'non-criminal lunatic' could remain in jail indefinitely. The question of transferring him to a mental hospital simply never came up.

Then how was a 'non-criminal lunatic' to get out of jail?

If and when a visiting psychiatrist decided that a patient had recovered, he certified him as medically fit. The case then went back to the magistrate who had originally sent the person to jail. This could take a while, especially if he had been picked up in a distant district. The process of discharge might take months. Murthy and Dhanda found that most patients at Alipore, many at Behrampore and Dum Dum, and a fair number at Presidency had been certified as medically fit. They were simply waiting to be released. Nobody knew when this would happen.

Not long after *Unlock the Padlock* was drafted, the Indian Lunacy Act was repealed. According to the new mental health law, a person could only be detained for observation under 'proper medical custody'. Evidently, this would rule out jails, sub-jails, and lock-ups.

In August 1993, the Supreme Court ruled that sending non-criminal mentally ill persons to jail was both illegal and unconstitutional. It ordered the West Bengal government to stop doing so at once. It asked the Calcutta High Court to suggest what could be done about the existing 'non-criminal lunatics' who needed treatment, and the ones who had recovered. And it directed the state government to improve mental health services, on the lines proposed by Murthy and Dhanda.

The court went one step further. It directed every state government to submit facts and figures about its institutions where the mentally ill were housed, its procedures for admission and discharge, its facilities for treatment and care, and its response to the recommendations made in the report of the two commissioners.

~

Meanwhile, magistrates in Assam continued to send 'non-criminal lunatics' to jail.

In May 1994, the Supreme Court appointed a commission to make sure that its eight-month old order was obeyed in Assam. Gopal Subramanium, a senior advocate in the Supreme Court, was given all of four weeks to do so.

On his arrival in Gauhati, Subramanium met the home secretary, who had apparently not heard of the Supreme Court's order. He then met the chief secretary and various senior officers. By this time he was convinced that the task could not be left to the bureaucracy. So he decided to take charge and conduct the proceedings 'totally like a judge'. First he got the home secretary to issue a circular to put a stop to sending 'non-criminal lunatics' to jail. Then he announced that he would personally interview every 'non-criminal lunatic' who was in jail at the time.

True to his word, the commissioner went from jail to jail. He took with him a psychiatrist, as well as officers from the district administration and the police. One by one, the prisoners came before the group. After studying the available records, Subramanium and the psychiatrist spoke with each person. Local officials were free to ask questions as well. The results were quite astonishing.

A few of the 'non-criminal lunatics' needed to be hospitalised, and a few were advised outpatient treatment. But the vast majority were, in fact, 'perfectly normal'. Oddly, many of these persons had been labelled as 'chronic schizophrenic'.

Had all these 'lunatics' been miraculously cured? Or had they been 'perfectly sane' to begin with?

The law allowed guardians of a mentally ill person to petition a magistrate for admission to a mental hospital. But the general practice in Assam was to go to the police instead. In 'strangely beautiful' handwritten applications that were 'suspiciously too similar', they stated that their ward was creating a nuisance, or threatening assault, or behaving dangerously. As 'good samaritans', the police would then assist the family 'out of compassion' and submit its application to a magistrate. The magistrate did not examine the person, nor did he call for a medical opinion. He simply ordered the person to be kept in jail 'until recovery'. But the jail did not provide regular psychiatric evaluation. Nor did it provide proper psychiatric treatment. In effect, a 'non-criminal lunatic' could be kept in jail indefinitely.

Subramanium figured that unscrupulous guardians, police, and magistrates were part of a 'vicious racket' to get rid of inconvenient persons who may or may not have been mentally ill. Unaware of what was going on, senior officers had remained in 'a blissful world of their own'.

As Gopal Subramanium was acting 'totally like a judge', he decided where each person should go after being released from jail. The seriously ill were to be admitted to a hospital for treatment. The destitute were to be taken to a home run by a social organisation. And the rest were to be sent back home.

Sending a person home was not as simple as it sounded. To make sure that he actually got there, Subramanium directed the superintendent of police to choose a competent officer as an escort. He also directed the district magistrate to make sure that there was enough fuel for the trip. But getting there was not enough. Relatives would have to agree to accept the person. Considering that they may have pushed him into jail in the first place, this could require some amount of persuasion. Subramanium took it upon himself to suggest how this might be done.

Halfway through this elaborate exercise, a bizarre fact came to light. Even before Subramanium had visited the first jail on his list, the authorities had surreptitiously released 141 'non-criminal lunatics'. Mere chance had prevented them from releasing the rest before Subramanium arrived on the spot to interview them. Denying that it had anything to do with this, the state government explained it away as a panic reaction of local officials. But, as Subramanium discovered, the government had indeed ordered the move. To cover its tracks, it had taken care to issue a verbal order rather than a written one. Magistrates had then sprung into action, doctors were called in, medical reports were readied, release orders were issued, and guardians were told to take their wards away. All this was done at top speed, and without the attention to detail that each individual case deserved.

The state government's attempt to scuttle the inquiry did not entirely succeed. Gopal Subramanium was able to arrange for the release of 225 persons in a thorough, transparent manner. His report documented the desperate plight of 'non-criminal lunatics', the lapses of individual officers, and the infirmities of the system. *Justicia Virtutum Regina* also suggested a wide range of measures to improve mental health services in Assam. The Supreme Court accepted the entire report and instructed the state government to act on it.

~

In 1993, the Supreme Court had struck down the jailing of 'non-criminal lunatics' as illegal and unconstitutional. This ruling would take effect slowly. By the year 2000, there were only 307 'non-criminal lunatics' in jail, and only in six states. West Bengal led with 120 persons. Assam had none. From 2001, the category vanished from official prison statistics. It was replaced by 'inmates suffering from mental illness', with separate figures for convicts, undertrials, detenus, and 'others'. Of the 1,420 such inmates reported that year, 53 per cent were undertrials and 39 per cent were convicts.

A 'criminal lunatic' could still be held indefinitely in jail, as well as in a mental hospital. Cases of this sort came up in court from time to time. Raghunandan Gope, Charanjeet Singh, and Machang Lalung were but three of the very many.

In December 1981, an article in the *Indian Express* reported that certain mentally ill prisoners had spent two to three decades in the Hazaribagh central jail. Based on this article, Veena Sethi wrote to the Supreme Court in January 1982, on behalf of the Hazaribagh Free Legal Aid Committee. When asked to respond, the Bihar government was ready with the details. One of the persons on the list was Raghunandan Gope, an undertrial. Accused of murder in 1950, he was incapable of standing trial at the time. Since then, there was no record of any medical examination, nor of any medical treatment. In January 1982, he was declared to be of sound mind, and capable of taking care of himself. It was impossible to say how long he had been this way. The Supreme Court decided that there was no point in prosecuting him, as he had already spent 32 years in jail. Raghunandan Gope was therefore released.

Charanjeet Singh was arrested for murder in 1985. Then 55 years old, he was suffering from schizophrenia and was unable to stand trial. In the absence of suitable treatment, his medical condition worsened. In 2002, the National Human Rights Commission took up his case. An article about the case in the *Hindustan Times* led Manisha Bhandari to petition the Delhi High Court. On the court's orders, he was then treated at various hospitals in the city. By this time, Charanjeet Singh was also suffering from senile dementia, renal failure, and cancer. The authorities tried to shift him out of Tihar jail to a halfway house or an old-age home. Given his state of health, this did not work out. Nor was it possible to release him on bail, because he had been deserted by his family. In March 2005, the court decided to drop the charges against Charanjeet Singh. Not just because he had already spent 20 years in jail, but also because he would never be capable of standing trial. With nowhere else to go, he was supposed to spend the rest of his days in a mental hospital.

Quite by chance, a visiting official from the National Human Rights Commission came across Machang Lalung working quietly in the garden at the Tezpur mental hospital in early

2005. Arrested in 1951 for causing grievous harm, Machang was brought to the hospital as an undertrial. In 1967, he was found fit to stand trial. However, no trial took place. He was no longer on any medication, and was no longer considered mentally ill. The maximum sentence for his alleged crime – whose records were untraceable – was 10 years. As he had already been in custody for 54 years, the commission sought his release.

Machang could not recall when or why he had been arrested. When he was taken to the vicinity of his village, he did not find the place familiar. So he was brought back to the hospital. Quite by chance, a man from his village came to the hospital for treatment. After he got home, this man asked around and was able to trace Machang's family. Apparently, Machang's close relatives had all passed away. But a niece remembered having been told about him. Eventually, he was identified on the basis of burn scars on his palms, and two missing fingers on his right hand.

On 1 July 2005, Machang was released on a personal bond of one rupee. The state government granted him a sum of Rs 300,000 as compensation, and a monthly stipend of Rs 1,000 for life.

In 2007, Assamese film-maker Aneisha Sharma won an award for *Freedom at the Edge* at the Boston International Film Festival. The documentary was based on the story of Machang Lalung.

Machung Lalung died later that year.

The insanity of institutions is more difficult to cure than the disorders of demented inmates. The finest investment in constitutional compassion is in transformation of mental health centres. But where is the wish, the will, the wisdom?[23]

---

[23] Prolegomenon by Justice V.R. Krishna Iyer, *Report of National Expert Committee on Women Prisoners* (New Delhi: Government of India, Ministry of Human Resource Development, Department of Women and Child Development, 1987), 14.

TWELVE

Hope for Hospitals

We have had occasions to see lunatic asylums in one or two States and we find that the conditions in these lunatic asylums are wholly revolting and one begins to wonder whether they are places for making insane persons sane or sane persons insane.[24]

By design, the mental hospital was cut off from the world outside its walls. Rumour and gossip apart, an outsider would rarely know what it was like on the inside. Its internal affairs would rarely be aired in any public forum. And while Justice D.A. Desai and Justice P.N. Bhagwati had actually seen a 'lunatic asylum' at close quarters, most judges would rarely have an occasion to do so.

In the early 1980s, the press began to offer the odd glimpse within mental hospitals. And public-spirited citizens began to ask the courts to intervene in the way they were run. Who were these extraordinary people? Most of them were lawyers, journalists, activists, or social workers. None were from the field of medicine.

---

[24] Supreme Court of India, *Mrs. Veena Sethi vs State of Bihar and Ors.*, order dated 11 May 1982, https://indiankanoon.org/doc/1928844/.

Prodded by press reports and petitions alike, the courts began to turn the spotlight on mental hospitals across the country.

~

In 1986, two residents of Patna, Rakesh Chandra Narayan and Subodh Chandra Narayan, wrote to the Chief Justice of India about the Bihar government's mental hospital at Kanke. Treating their letter as a public interest petition, the Supreme Court got the district's chief judicial magistrate to take a look.

The magistrate reported 'shocking' and 'savage' conditions that resembled those of a 'medieval torture house'. The hospital had only 300 beds for its 1,580 patients. Several patients slept on the bare floor. No ward had proper doors and windows. Broken cots were propped up to prevent escape. Electric lights did not work. The patients were in total darkness from dusk to dawn. None of the fans worked either. Toilets were choked. Patients were forced to relieve themselves in an adjacent open field. Some patients were naked, others wore torn clothes. Insect bites were clearly visible on their bodies. There was an acute shortage of water. Clothes were washed just once in four to six weeks. Around 300 patients were no longer mentally ill. They continued to live on the premises. Among the 13 'cured' convicts, one had been at Kanke since 1947.

The medical facilities were no better. Of the 16 posts for medical officers, as many as seven lay vacant. The hospital was headed by an acting medical superintendent who lacked 'adequate control' over colleagues and staff. Several doctors were absent for days on end. On one of his visits, the magistrate found no doctors on duty. Yet the attendance register showed them as present. Equipment and instruments were defective. There was no refrigerator to store lifesaving drugs. And no inventory of medical supplies. Several patients claimed that they had not been given any medicine for many months.

The court asked the government of Bihar for an explanation. The government said that it was aware of the situation and would act in the coming months. This did not reassure the court. In October 1986, it ordered the government to act 'forthwith' to fix the obvious flaws. For instance, the budget for food – then pegged at Rs 3 per patient per day – must go up to Rs 10. The ceiling on spending on medicines – then a sum of Rs 1.90 per patient per day – must be scrapped. 'Pure' drinking water must be supplied. Sanitary conditions must be restored in lavatories and bathrooms. All patients must be given beds, mattresses, and blankets. A qualified psychiatrist must be appointed. And so must a medical superintendent.

Over the next two years, more facts came out, and more explanations were filed. In September 1988, the court switched to a more drastic line. Justice Ranganath Misra observed that though the government was aware of the 'sordid situation', it had failed to comply with the court's directions. He noted its 'general lethargy' in 'rising from slumber', and the absence of 'appropriate sincerity in action'. He therefore decided that the hospital would no longer be run directly by the state department of health. Instead, it would be under a committee chaired by a sitting judge of the Patna High Court. This committee was expected to remove the defects in the hospital. It was also expected to figure out how to transform it into a modern scientific institution.

Managed by the committee and monitored by the court, things began to move. In 1994, the hospital was registered under the Societies Act. It would still be funded and staffed by the state government. But its new managing committee would have considerable control over finance and administration.

From then onwards, the hospital did not look back. It had taken eight years of judicial oversight to drag it out of the woods.

Kanke was not the only mental hospital to be hauled up in court. The list included Agra, Calicut, Delhi, Gwalior, Mankundu, Panjim, Tezpur, Trichur, Trivandrum, and Yeravda. These cases were often similar, but their outcome tended to vary.

Together with a persistent petitioner, a committed court could open up the hospital to scrutiny. It could bring in independent experts from the fields of medicine, administration, and law. It could issue orders to the authorities and set deadlines for them to act. And it could keep a case open – for years – till it was satisfied with the outcome. If a state government chose to cooperate, this outcome could be quite dramatic. The hospital could get more attention and more resources. It could obtain better facilities and offer better services. And – like the mental hospitals at Agra, Delhi, Gwalior, Kanke, and Tezpur – it could get greater freedom to function.

Yet public interest litigation did not always lead to a dramatic outcome. Nor did it result in an overhaul of the system. Even as the judiciary was quick to step into the turf of the executive, it skirted that of the legislature. Court rulings did not highlight the flaws in the mental health law. Nor did they secure the constitutional rights of the mentally ill.

⁓

The Constitution of India had been adopted on 26 January 1950. It was the result of deliberation and discussion in the Constituent Assembly of India over a period of three years. Elsewhere, the United Nations was engaged in defining its own position on human rights. India was one of the 18 countries whose delegates drafted this document. Three Indian delegates – Vijay Lakshmi Pandit, Hansa Mehta, and M.R. Masani – happened to be members of the constituent assembly. In fact, both Mehta and Masani were on its panel on fundamental rights.

The Universal Declaration of Human Rights was adopted by the United Nations General Assembly on 10 December 1948. This declaration did not merely reflect the international outlook at the time. It also reflected India's resolve as an independent, sovereign nation.

The United Nations' position on human rights would later become more explicit in two separate treaties. One was on civil and political rights. The other was on economic, social, and cultural rights. Unlike the universal declaration, these treaties were binding, and no country could enter into them lightly. Both were opened for signature in 1966. Both needed the consent of 35 members to take effect. Both did so in 1976.

At that point, India was under a state of national emergency, and its citizens' civil rights had been suspended. It was hardly in a position to ratify either treaty. The Emergency was lifted in 1977. India ratified the two treaties in 1979. But it would struggle to comply with their demands.

Over much of the 1980s, the border states of Assam and Punjab were racked by secessionist insurgency. By the end of the decade, Jammu and Kashmir was in turmoil too. As the government tried to quell these movements by the use of force, it was accused – at home and abroad – of widespread human rights violations. India was particularly sensitive to criticism on Kashmir, a region that was extremely vulnerable to external intervention.

In 1991, the government had launched radical economic reforms, for which it sought the support of the international community. This was not a good time to draw flak for its human rights record. In 1993, it set up the National Human Rights Commission – a statutory body that was designed in line with the latest global standards. This was India's first big step to promote and protect its citizens' constitutional right to life, liberty, equality, and dignity.

The National Human Rights Commission had plenty on its plate. It took a while to turn its attention to the state of mental hospitals across the country. One of the first things it did was to sponsor a country-wide survey by the National Institute of Mental Health and Neurosciences, Bangalore. The report of this survey was published in 1999.

The survey pointed out that each of India's 37 public mental hospitals had a peculiar history of its own. A third of them actually dated back to the 19th century, while others came up later. Even though old hospitals had been given new names over the years, some held on to their old structures. Fourteen of them were built like jails. The one at Murshidabad had, in fact, been a jail till 1980. Old wards at Vizagapatam were like jail cells with iron gates. Both old and new wards at Trichur had iron bars and gates.

Maintenance was exceptionally bad at 26 hospitals. Leaking roofs, overflowing toilets, eroded floors, and broken doors and windows were common sights. Old buildings at Amritsar, Indore, Nagpur, and Thane were only fit to be demolished. Certain wards at Tezpur were unliveable. The walls of Murshidabad's wards were crawling with lice. Vizagapatam's wards stood out for their cobwebs, mosquitoes, and foul stench.

Half the hospitals had only closed wards, where patients were kept locked for much of the day. Sixteen had small cells where patients remained confined alone or in a group. Many cells did not have water, beds, bedding, or toilets. At Indore,

                    Daman Singh

most male patients were kept in cells, and many of them were chained. At Vizagapatam, patients were often left in a cell with their hands and feet tied. Sometimes they injured themselves by repeatedly banging their head against the iron bars. Plates of food were pushed through these bars. At Calicut, a large number of patients were squeezed into cells meant for one person. There was not enough room for them to lie down. They ate from plates that were placed on the floor outside the bars of the cell. At Benares, new patients spent their first two weeks locked up in a small cell without light, water, bedding, or a toilet. During this period they received no treatment. In the overcrowded cells at Trichur, patients were stripped down to their underwear. This was supposed to prevent them from using their clothing to strangle themselves.

In the past, overcrowding was a common problem. But this was no longer the case. Only four hospitals were overfull – Calicut and Trivandrum overwhelmingly so. A few wards in various other hospitals were also overcrowded.

On an average, about a third of all patients slept on the floor. Indore provided patients with metal beds without mattresses, pillows, or sheets. Cement blocks served as beds in certain wards at Gwalior. Most hospitals had enough fans. But none had heating, even during severely cold winters. Fourteen hospitals had poor lighting. Some of these reported cases of assault, robbery, and rape.

Thirteen hospitals had very dirty toilets. Some were choked with faeces. Dharwar's toilets and bathrooms did not have running water. Neither did toilets at Hyderabad, Jamnagar, Nagpur, and Thane. Most women's toilets at Indore did not have doors. Male patients at Ahmedabad and Indore urinated and defecated in open drains. One of the women's wards at Gwalior had no toilets at all. Its walls were smeared with faecal matter. Most wards at Murshidabad had human excreta on the floor.

Not every hospital had safe drinking water. A bucket of water was often placed outside the ward. Patients would reach through the bars, fill up a mug, and drink straight from it. They shared this mug with the rest of the ward. The quality of food varied across hospitals. So did the daily budget for food. This was as generous as Rs 30 per patient in Assam and Bihar, and as meagre as Rs 5 per patient in Tamil Nadu.

Random facts added to the bleak findings of the survey. Twelve hospitals did not allow patients to be visited by family members. Twenty-six shaved the head of all male patients. Seventeen did this to women patients. Children were admitted to closed wards at Vizagapatam and Yeravda. Undertrials at Benares spent long years at the hospital as police personnel were rarely available to escort them to court hearings. At Thane, patients who had recovered were housed together with those who had not. About 80 patients escaped from Kanke each year by climbing a tree and jumping over the boundary wall. Incidents of drunken behaviour and assault by attendants were common at Madras. Attendants at Agra used a long stick to control patients. Passers-by could peer into the women's wards at Indore.

Medical facilities were a mixed bag. Gwalior did not have a psychiatrist. Nor did Jamnagar. Elsewhere, a psychiatrist was expected to treat from 10 to over 200 patients. Four hospitals had no nurses. Fifteen did not have a clinical psychologist. Twelve did not have a social worker. Fifteen did not have emergency medical facilities. Seven lacked a laboratory for routine investigations.

Drug therapy and electroconvulsive therapy were the standard lines of psychiatric treatment. In general, anaesthesia and muscle relaxants were advised to make electroconvulsive therapy more safe and less traumatic. However, only half the hospitals followed this advice. Thirteen offered no psychotherapy. Few provided competent occupational therapy. Patients had little or no recreation in most hospitals. Rehabilitation programmes were also rare.

In short, a number of mental hospitals were a lot like 19th century lunatic asylums.

While the survey dwelt on the defects of the mental hospitals, it also brought out their achievements. In this arena, the National Institute of Mental Health and Neurosciences was clearly way ahead. Six other hospitals were also 'relatively good'. Of these, Kanke and Tezpur were more or less autonomous. Ranchi was under the central government. Only three hospitals run by state governments made the cut – Delhi, Jammu, and Panjim.

In the years that followed, committees were appointed, conferences were organised, workshops were held, guidelines were framed, proposals were sanctioned, projects were executed, and better practices were put in place.

By 2008, these efforts had begun to pay off. Change was visible almost everywhere, even in hospitals that were earlier listed as 'very poor'. Amritsar, for instance, was no longer run directly by the department of health. Like many medical institutions in the state, it now came under the Punjab Health System Corporation. It had a brand new building, with a modern kitchen, a mechanised laundry, and a sewage treatment plant. Each ward had a suitable arrangement for drinking water, beds and bedding, toilets and bathrooms, and geysers for hot water baths. Most wards had a television set as well. The hospital had stopped giving electroconvulsive treatment without anaesthesia and muscle relaxants. It had also stopped tying up its patients.

Nudged along by the National Human Rights Commission, a system to reform India's mental hospitals was finally taking shape.

These reforms, however, were not backed by the law on mental health.

~

On 13 December 2006, the United Nations General Assembly had adopted the Convention on the Rights of People with Disabilities. This treaty defined disability as a long-term physical, mental, intellectual, or sensory impairment. It affirmed that all persons with disabilities were entitled to the same human rights and fundamental freedoms as other persons. It explained these rights, and spelt out how they ought to apply. And it called upon member states to uphold these rights in their respective laws, policies, programmes, and procedures. The treaty opened for signature in March 2007, and took effect in May 2008. India was one of the first countries to ratify it.

India already had a law on the rights of persons with disabilities. This, however, would have to be amended. In 2009, the ministry of social justice set about doing so. It also informed the ministry of health that the law on mental health would have to be amended too. The ministry of health took up the matter in early 2010.

As both sides got to work, they took different positions on the rights of the mentally ill. The 'social welfare side' argued for uniform clauses for all aspects of all kinds of disability. On the other hand, the 'health side' called for separate clauses for the medical treatment of mental illness. Eventually, the latter would prevail.

Two fresh laws were thus enacted – the Rights of Persons with Disability Act in 2016, and the Mental Healthcare Act in 2017. Both conformed to the Convention on the Rights of People with Disabilities.

The Mental Healthcare Act had been prompted by India's need to fulfil its international obligations. But it actually did very much more. It made it mandatory for the government to provide suitable mental healthcare and services. And it crafted a legal framework for this to be done.

The new law broke away from the prescriptions of the past. It defined mental illness as a medical condition that demanded scientific diagnosis and treatment. For the purpose of treatment, it viewed allopathy as one among several systems of medicine. But the law did not take a purely medical line. It also covered patients' care and their eventual rehabilitation. Thus, psychiatrists, clinical psychologists, mental health nurses, and psychiatric social workers were each to be represented in regulatory bodies at the district, state, and central level. Strikingly, so too were non-government organisations, care-givers, and mentally ill persons themselves.

A new system to regulate mental health institutions was the linchpin of the new law. It brought into its fold all the institutions – public and private, general and specialist – that were engaged in providing inpatient services to those who were mentally ill. These inpatient services included treatment, care, and rehabilitation. The mental hospital was but one of the flock. It was meant to be turned to only as a last resort.

In a radical step forward, the new law presumed that a mentally ill person had the capacity to decide on all matters related to his treatment and care. Even so, it recognised that this capacity could vary from person to person, and from time to time. Under the new law, a patient's informed consent was required for all relevant decisions. But if and when his capacity was found to be diminished, he was supposed to be assisted by a duly authorised representative.

What did these changes mean for the mental hospital?

They meant that the hospital was bound to uphold the human rights and fundamental freedoms of its patients. It was bound to provide quality medical treatment and patient care. It was bound to meet the minimum standards that were laid down by regulatory bodies. It was bound to follow a formal procedure to assess a patient's capacity, and to obtain his informed consent – at the time of admission, during treatment and care, and at discharge. It was also bound to prepare him for the world outside its walls.

Simply put, the mental hospital would have to become a modern medical institution for specialist treatment and care of the mentally ill.

> The promise of India's Mental Healthcare Act, 2017, … will remain just that – a promise – without effective implementation of the legislation. Readers who are not familiar with India will be more than a little surprised by the idea of a law existing on statute but not being implemented. However, India has a history of enacting progressive social sector legislation which remains unimplemented and 'customary practices' continue unhindered.

> … [The Act's] mandate is mammoth and far-reaching in terms of the obligations on the central and state governments to ensure the right to access mental healthcare and treatment. The success of this mandate will depend entirely on how all mental health stakeholders can be motivated to actualize commitments made under this law, and, further, how proactive civil society is in compelling governments to fulfil this mandate.[25]

---

[25] Soumitra Pathare and Arjun Kapoor, 'Implementation Update on Mental Healthcare Act, 2017', in *India's Mental Healthcare Act, 2017: Building laws, Protecting Rights*, by R.M. Duffy and B.D. Kelly (Singapore: Springer Nature Singapore Pte Ltd, 2020), 251, 263.

THIRTEEN

Are We There Yet?

In the face of that desperation, patients endure hours in the hospital's dirty halls for a five-minute audience in the presence of a dozen other patients and their accompanying relatives. This is not a population given to seeking treatment for psychiatric problems. In fact, mental illness carries a heavy stigma, which explains why most patients opt to see Dr. Hussain at the general hospital rather than the psychiatric ward. His resources are so stretched that some people get a single, cursory session, with little or no follow-up. The only thing in generous supply is medication, which the beleaguered staff hand out like Tootsie Rolls at Halloween.[26]

When it comes to maladies of the mind, there is an enduring culture in the Indian subcontinent of turning to the occult, to faith, and to traditional methods of healing. In the 18th century, another option was added to this list – the lunatic asylum. The asylum was meant to protect society from the disturbing, disruptive, and possibly dangerous influence of the insane. It was a primitive form of captivity in cruel and barbaric conditions.

---

[26] Judith Matloff and Robert Neckelsberg, 'Beyond the Breaking Point', Dart Center for Journalism and Trauma, 9 April 2009, https://dartcenter.org/content/beyond-breaking-point.

The first officially recognised – though privately run – asylum was established in Calcutta in the year 1788. Soon enough, public asylums came up across the breadth of British India. Foreign in both concept and design, the asylum became the approved place to confine the insane.

By the middle of the 19th century, medical science was thinking differently about insanity. The origin of this affliction was not yet clear. And its antidote was not yet known. But there was reason to believe that it could be corrected through humane and therapeutic treatment. As this view took root in the Western world, asylums began to be refashioned as institutions for the care of the mentally ill. While Britain had been quick to attend to its own asylums, it took a while to turn to those in its largest colony.

British India's story of asylum reform began in the early 20th century. The original plan was to gradually replace small mental hospitals with large ones that were better designed and better run. Each large mental hospital was to be placed under a full-time medical specialist. This specialist was expected to modernise the treatment and care of the mentally ill.

The plan took off well. Bit by bit, new ideas found a foothold in the large hospitals that were led by specialists. But small mental hospitals continued to exist in much the same manner as before. Mental illness was not seen as a public health priority. Local governments had all sorts of views of their own. Funds proved to be elusive. And qualified personnel were hard to get. Without a unified policy on mental healthcare, the spread of modern ideas was destined to be fragmented. And while all the asylums had been readily baptised as mental hospitals, only a few lived up to their new name.

Independent India thus inherited both decent mental hospitals and decrepit ones. It also inherited all the impediments that had interrupted their reform. As these were tackled in fits and starts, the gains were slight and slow. Makers of public policy did not root for an overhaul of the system. And neither did public authorities.

The push for change would come from the courts and from the press. By the early 1990s, the call for course correction was loud as well as clear. This led to various improvements in the way a number of mental hospitals were run. But major mental healthcare reform in the country would still have to wait.

Ultimately, the insistence for major reform came from the global community. In a series of resolutions and binding treaties, the United Nations had set out the rights of the mentally ill, and the principles of institutional treatment and care. When India's government was confronted with its inescapable international obligations, it finally took the plunge.

The story of major mental healthcare reform in independent India thus began in the early 21st century.

There is, today, an aspirational mental healthcare law, a progressive national mental health policy, and an ambitious national mental health programme. Serious efforts are underway to transform mental hospitals into modern medical institutions. A lengthy stay in such an institution is no longer considered necessary, nor is it seen as desirable. And mental hospitals no longer have the sole prerogative to treat the mentally ill. Psychiatry has thus travelled from mental hospitals to general hospitals, and from inpatient wards to outpatient clinics.

As a branch of medical science, psychiatry deals with the symptoms of mental illness. But it does not always have all the answers. Several are furnished by disciplines that look behind symptoms, and beyond them as well. Clinical psychologists, counsellors, occupational therapists, and psychiatric social workers are some of the other specialists who can enable a person to find – and to follow – a path that leads to a meaningful life.

Yet, four out of five mentally ill persons in India go untreated. Why is that so?

For millions of people across the country, a mental health specialist – of any kind – is either unknown, unavailable, or unaffordable. With just one specialist to a population of fifty thousand, this is not surprising. It is tempting to pin the blame on the woes of a developing country struggling to shake off a colonial legacy of neglect. But most countries in the same income bracket as India have actually done way better. And plenty among them have, in fact, a history of foreign occupation, despotic regimes, and civil war.

In a society riddled with ignorance and prejudice, mental illness is still poorly understood. There is still a tendency to ignore or to dismiss disturbing feelings, thoughts, and behaviour that recur or persist over time. And to overlook what could lie behind unexplained physical ailments that refuse to go away. These symptoms might not even be recognised by a general medical practitioner, let alone by family and friends. And ascribing them to mental illness summons up the spectre of denial and of shame.

Mental illness can devastate, disable, and demean the person whom it besets. It can also put the family through crushing emotional and economic strain. Even where mental health services exist, accessing them takes time as well as money. Should substantial home care be required, this is an added cost to bear. And coping with social stigma takes a toll of its own.

What happens to thousands of persons who desperately need the support that their family cannot – or will not – provide? These persons exist on the margins of society, invisible and unheard. In countless homes they live without dignity and decency, with no hope of a better life. They remain unclaimed in the wards of mental hospitals – institutions that are increasingly reluctant to retain patients merely because they have nowhere else to go. They are found in dubious facilities that either claim to cure, or else promise proper care. They wind up in shelters for beggars and for the destitute. And they fend for themselves on the streets, where deprivation and abuse is the order of the day.

The past tells us how the state chose to overlook opportunities to commit public policy and public resources to mental healthcare. It also tells us how society chose to turn its back on its mentally ill. If the future is to be any different, the state and society must find the resolve to do enormously more, and enormously better.

No, we are not there yet. We are just about getting started.

Mental illness is closer to us than we realize. Let us take a close look around our own lives – our family, relatives, friends, colleagues, people who live in our neighbourhood … In the criss-cross of these networks we will find someone with a mental illness: an aging relative, perhaps, who suffers from dementia, a neighbour's son who is so afraid of crowds that he hardly ever leaves home; a colleague's young daughter who committed suicide; a friend who has extreme mood swings; a co-worker's grandmother who suffers from acute anxiety … And what about ourselves?[27]

---

[27] Tata Trusts, *Pathways of Hope: Stories of Courage; a Journey in Mental Health and Wellness* (Mumbai: Sir Dorabji Tata Trust, 2017), 163.

Sources

1. Asylum

Annual Reports of lunatic asylums in Assam, Bengal, Bombay, Central Provinces, Madras, North-Western Provinces and Oudh, and Punjab for the year 1900.

Anon. 'Medical Progress in India during the Past Century'. *Indian Medical Gazette*, vol. 36, no. 1 (January 1901): 21–24.

Ewens, G.F.W. *Insanity in India: Its Symptoms and Diagnosis; with Reference to the Relation of Crime and Insanity.* Calcutta: Thacker, Spink & Co., 1908.

2. The New Era

Anon. 'Asylums in India'. *The Journal of Mental Science,* vol. XLV, no. 191 (October 1899): 765–767.

Fraser, A.H.L., and C.J.H. Warden. Note on asylum administration, dated 7 August 1894. Proposed improvements in the administration of lunatic asylums in India. Home department/ Medical branch, File no. 97–99, March 1895. National Archives of India.

Hewett, J.P. Letter to local governments, dated 29 March 1895. Proposed improvements in the administration of lunatic asylums in India. Home department/ Medical branch, File no. 97–99, March 1895. National Archives of India.

Lodge Patch, C.J. *A Critical Review of the Punjab Mental Hospital from 1840 to 1930*. Lahore: Punjab Government Record Office Publications, 1931.

McDowall, T.W. 'The Insane in India and their Treatment'. *The Journal of Mental Science*, vol. XLIII, no. 183 (October 1897): 683–702.

Rice, W.R. Memorandum on asylum administration, dated 21 February 1895. Proposed improvements in the administration of lunatic asylums in India. Home department/ Medical branch, File no. 97–99, March 1895. National Archives of India.

______. Note dated 17 September 1894. Proposed improvements in the administration of lunatic asylums in India. Home department/ Medical branch, File no. 97–99, March 1895. National Archives of India.

______. Note dated 24 October 1894. Proposed improvements in the administration of lunatic asylums in India. Home department/ Medical branch, File no. 97–99, March 1895. National Archives of India.

Shaw, W.S.J. 'Some Generalisations on the Scope, Construction and Administration of Central Asylums in India'. *The Indian Medical Gazette*, vol. 49, no. 11 (November 1914): 424–427.

Summary of the responses to J.P. Hewett's letter of 29 March 1894 from local governments, dated 1 October 1896. Administration of lunatic asylums in India. Home department/ Medical branch, File no. 188–232, August 1897. National Archives of India.

Triennial Report on the Lunatic Asylums in Bengal for the Years 1903, 1904 and 1905. Calcutta: the Bengal Secretariat Book Depot, 1906.

3. World War 1

Annual and Triennial Reports of lunatic asylums in Assam (1912–19), Bengal (1900–24), Bihar and Orissa (1918–19, 1925), Bombay (1900–19), Central Provinces (1911–19), Madras (1900–19), Punjab (1900–19), and United Province of Agra & Oudh (and former North-Western Provinces and Oudh; 1900–19).

Anon. 'Service and War Notes'. *The Indian Medical Gazette*, vol. 50, no. 2 (February 1915): 75–80.

Hehir, Patrick. *The Medical Profession in India*. London: Henry Frowde and Hodder & Stoughton, 1923.

Shaw, W.S.J. 'Some Generalisations on the Scope, Construction and Administration of Central Asylums in India'. *The Indian Medical Gazette*, vol. 49, no. 11 (November 1914): 424–437.

4. The Alienists

Annual Report on the Working of the Indian Mental Hospital, Kanke, in Bihar and Orissa for the Year 1930. Patna: Superintendent, Government Printing, 1932.

Annual Report on the Working of the Indian Mental Hospital, Kanke, in Bihar and Orissa for the Year 1936. Patna: Superintendent, Government Printing, 1938.

Berkeley-Hill, Owen A. R. 'A Plea for the Inception of a Mental Hygiene Movement in India'. *The Indian Medical Gazette*, vol. 58, no. 6 (June 1923): 242–244.

Das, Banarsi. 'A Psychiatric Tour of Europe'. *The Indian Medical Gazette*, vol. 66, no. 9 (September 1931): 517–518.

Hehir, Patrick. *The Medical Profession in India*. London: Henry Frowde and Hodder & Stoughton, 1923.

Overbeck-Wright, A. Note on the alienist department in India, dated 5 January 1919. DGIMS/ Medical section/ IMD, File no. 502, April 1918. National Archives of India.

Shaw, W.S.J. Letter to the personal assistant to the Surgeon-General, Government of Bombay, Poona, dated 16 July 1920. Amendment of the Indian Lunacy Act, 1912 (IV of 1912) so as to provide for the change of designation of lunatic asylums to mental hospitals: inter-provincial recovery of charges for maintenance of lunatics; and the management of the Ranchi European Mental Hospital by a board of trustees. Question of further amending the Act so as to provide for 'Urgency Orders'. Home department/ Jails branch, File no. 88, 1922. National Archives of India.

Statement of objects and reasons for amending the Indian Lunacy Act, dated 28 January 1922. Amendment of the Indian Lunacy Act, 1912 (IV of 1912) so as to provide for the change of designation of lunatic asylums to mental hospitals: inter-provincial recovery of charges for maintenance of lunatics; and the management of the Ranchi European Mental Hospital by a board of trustees. Question of further amending the Act so as to provide for 'Urgency Orders'. Home department/ Jails branch, File no. 88, 1922. National Archives of India.

Triennial Report on the Working of the Indian Mental Hospital, Kanke, in Bihar and Orissa for the Years 1930–32. Patna: Superintendent, Government Printing, 1933.

5. Bending the Rules

Annual Report on the Lunatic Asylums of Bengal for the Year 1900. Calcutta: Bengal Secretariat Press, 1901.

Annual Report on the Working of the Mental Hospitals in the Madras Presidency for the Year 1938. Madras: Superintendent, Government Press, 1939.

Ewens, G.F.W. *Insanity in India: Its Symptoms and Diagnosis, with Reference to the Relation of Crime and Insanity*. Calcutta: Thacker, Spink & Co., 1908.

Heffernan, P. 'The Voluntary Boarder'. *The Indian Medical Gazette* (November 1912): 433–435.

Letter from the Secretary of the European Association to the Home Secretary, Government of India, dated 9 October 1920. Amendment of the Indian Lunacy Act, 1912 (IV of 1912) so as to provide for the change of designation of lunatic asylums to mental hospitals: inter-provincial recovery of charges for maintenance of lunatics; and the management of the Ranchi European Mental Hospital by a board of trustees. Question of further amending the Act so as to provide for 'Urgency Orders'. Home department/ Jails branch, File no. 88, 1922. National Archives of India.

Lodge Patch, C.J. 'A Century of Psychiatry in the Punjab'. *The Journal of Mental Science*, vol. 85, no. 356 (May 1939): 381–391.

———. *A Critical Review of the Punjab Mental Hospital from 1840 to 1930*. Lahore: Punjab Government Record Office Publications, 1931.

Report on the European Hospital for Mental Diseases at Ranchi, for the Year 1927. Patna: Superintendent, Government Printing, Bihar and Orissa, 1929.

'Resolution Re Mental Defectives'. *The Council of State Debates*, vol. V (20 January–26 March 1925): 228–241.

Statistical Returns of the Lunatic Asylums in the Madras Presidency for the Year 1914. Madras: Superintendent, Government Press, 1915.

Triennial Report on the Working of the Punjab Lunatic Asylum for the Years 1909, 1910 and 1911. Lahore: Punjab Government Press, 1912.

6. Trends in Treatment

Annual and Triennial Reports of lunatic asylums/ mental hospitals in British India (1900–47).

Annual Report on the Working of the Ranchi Indian Mental Hospital, Kanke, in Bihar and Orissa, for the Year 1934. Patna: Superintendent, Government Printing, Bihar and Orissa, 1935.

Govindaswamy, M.V. 'Mental Disorder in India – a Review and a Prospect'. *The Indian Journal of Social Work*, vol. 7, no. 1 (1946): 41–48.

7. Legacy of the Raj

Annual and Triennial Reports of lunatic asylums/ mental hospitals in British India (1900–47).

Govindaswamy, M.V. 'Mental Disorder in India – a Review and a Prospect (Since 1946)'. *Indian Journal of Social Work*, vol. 9, no. 2 (1948): 96–104.

Report of the Health Survey and Development Committee, volume I, II
and III. Delhi: Manager of Publications, Government of India,
1946.

Note: In this chapter, mental hospital statistics for the year 1946 do not
include the Sir Cowasji Jehangir Mental Hospital in Hyderabad (Sind).
Figures for the Ranchi Indian Mental Hospital, Kanke, are for the year
1940–41. Figures for the European Mental Hospital at Ranchi are for
the year 1945–46.

8. Lahore

*Agreements Between India and Pakistan Reached at Inter-Dominion
Conferences held at New Delhi in Dec. 1948, Calcutta in April
1948, and Karachi in May 1948, and Some Related Documents.*
Delhi: Ministry of External Affairs and Commonwealth
Relations, Government of India, 1949.
*Annual Report of the Working of Punjab Mental Hospital, Amritsar, for
1949.* Simla: Controller of Printing and Stationery, Punjab,
1951.
*Annual Report of the Working of Punjab Mental Hospital, Amritsar, for
the Year 1950.*
*Annual Report of the Working of the Punjab Mental Hospital, Lahore, for
the Year 1949.* Lahore: Superintendent, Government Printing,
Punjab.
*Annual Report on the Working of Punjab Mental Hospital, Amritsar, for
the Year 1951.*
*Annual Report on the Working of the Punjab Mental Hospital, Lahore, for
the Year 1950.* Lahore: Superintendent, Government Printing,
West Pakistan, 1956.
*Annual Report on the Working of the Punjab Mental Hospital, Lahore, for
the Year 1951.* Lahore: Superintendent, Government Printing,
West Pakistan, 1956.
*Annual Report on the Working of the West Punjab Mental Hospital,
Lahore, 1947.* Lahore: Superintendent, Government Printing,
West Punjab, 1949.

Anon. 'Patients who Died in Lahore Mental Hospital'. *The Sunday Tribune*, 22 October 1950.

'Exchange of Mental Diseases Patients'. *Parliamentary Debates, Part 1 – Questions and Answers*, vol. VII (2 April–16 May 1951): 2907.

Khosla, Gopal Das. *Stern Reckoning: A Survey of the Events Leading up to and Following the Partition of India*. Delhi: Oxford University Press, 1989.

Rao, U. Bhaskar. *The Story of Rehabilitation*. Delhi: Department of Rehabilitation, Ministry of Labour, Employment and Rehabilitation, Government of India, 1967.

Report on the Working of the Punjab Mental Hospital, Lahore, for the Year 1948. Lahore: Superintendent, Government Printing, Punjab, 1950.

Walia, Varinder. '59 Years Later, He is Still Here'. *The Tribune* (Chandigarh), 26 October 2007.

9. Bringing Out a Bill

Central Intelligence Agency. 'A 1964 View of KGB Methods: Soviet Use of Assassination and Kidnapping'. [CIA memorandum prepared in February 1964 for The President's Commission on the Assassination of President Kennedy (The Warren Commission) and declassified in 1971]. https://carnegieendowment.org/files/SovietUseOfAssassination.pdf.

'Constitution of an All-India Mental Health Service'. *Rajya Sabha Official Debates, Part I – Question and Answer* (13 March 1961): 2538–2540. http://rsdebate.nic.in/handle/123456789/557924.

'C.P.W.D. Employee in Mental Hospital, Agra'. *Rajya Sabha Official Debates, Part I – Question and Answer* (24 August 1960): 1998–2002. http://rsdebate.nic.in/handle/123456789/560747.

'Inadequacy of Psychiatric Treatment Facilities'. *Lok Sabha Debates*, vol. IV, no. 21 (11 April 1985): 10–15.

'Lunatic Asylums'. *Lok Sabha Debates*, vol. LI, no. 13 (3 March 1966): 3571–3572.

'Mental Ailments in Service Personnel'. *Rajya Sabha Official Debates, Part 1 – Question and Answer* (25 August 1953): 125–128. http://rsdebate.nic.in/handle/123456789/588797.

'Mental Diseases in Army'. *Lok Sabha Debates*, vol. V, no. 44 (13 June 1962): 10541–10542.

'Mental Health Bill – continued'. *Lok Sabha Debates*, vol. XIII, no. 33 (7 April 1978): 356–392.

'Mental Health Bill'. *Lok Sabha Debates*, vol. XI, no. 23 (23 March 1978): 304–326.

'Pakistan Flag over Daulatabad Fort'. *Parliamentary Debates, Official Report, Part I – Questions and Answers*, vol. VI (23 February 1951): 1686–1687.

'Pilot Survey on Health of Workers in Rourkela Steel Plant'. *Lok Sabha Debates*, vol. XXXVIII, no. 22 (24 March 1970): 253–254.

'Plan for Mental Health Education and Protection of Mental Health at Grassroot Level'. *Lok Sabha Debates*, vol. IV, no. 26 (18 April 1985): 208–209.

'Preventive Detention (Second Amendment) Bill'. *Parliamentary Debates, House of the People, Official Report, Part II – Proceedings other than Questions and Answers*, vol. 1 (18 July 1952): 4070–4204.

'Professor Zelenovsky'. *Lok Sabha Debates*, vol. XI, no. 2 (11 February 1958): 67–68.

'Question of Privilege'. *Lok Sabha Debates*, vol. III, no. 1 (15 July 1957): 3535–3539.

'Question of Privilege'. *Lok Sabha Debates*, vol. V, no. 22 (12 August 1957): 7992–7993.

'Resolution re Sterilisation of Adults Suffering from Incurable Diseases or Insanity'. *Rajya Sabha Official Debates, Part 2 – Other than Question and Answer* (11 September 1953): 1924–1956. http://rsdebate.nic.in/handle/123456789/588223.

'Resolution re Sterilisation of Adults Suffering from Incurable Diseases or Insanity'. *Rajya Sabha Official Debates, Part 2 – Other than Question and Answer* (28 August 1953): 533–649. http://rsdebate.nic.in/handle/123456789/588290.

Sharma, Shridhar. *Mental Hospitals in India*. New Delhi: Directorate General of Health Services, Government of India, 1990.

'Statement referred to in reply to part (a) of starred question no. 634 regarding complacency of the State Governments in regard to mental diseases in India, answered by the Minister of Health' [on 28 March 1963; copy placed in Parliament Library, ref. no. LT-1042/ 63].

'Sterilisation of the Unfit Bill'. *Parliamentary Debates, House of the People, Official Report, Part I – Questions and Answers*, vol. 1 (30 July 1952): 4871–4896.

'Sterilisation of the Unfit Bill, 1964 – continued'. *Rajya Sabha Official Debates, Part 2 – Other than Question and Answer* (14 March 1969): 3804–3818. http://rsdebate.nic.in/handle/123456789/501806.

'Sterilisation of the Unfit Bill, 1964 – continued'. *Rajya Sabha Official Debates, Part 2 – Other than Question and Answer* (20 March 1970): 145–183. http://rsdebate.nic.in/handle/123456789/488613.

'Sterilisation of the Unfit Bill, 1964 – continued'. *Rajya Sabha Official Debates, Part 2 – Other than Question and Answer* (27 February 1969): 1812–1858. http://rsdebate.nic.in/handle/123456789/502048.

'Sterilisation of the Unfit Bill, 1964 – continued'. *Rajya Sabha Official Debates, Part 2 – Other than Question and Answer* (27 February 1969): 1859–1880. http://rsdebate.nic.in/handle/123456789/502056.

'Sterilisation of the Unfit Bill, 1964 – continued'. *Rajya Sabha Official Debates, Part 2 – Other than Question and Answer* (28 November 1969): 2035–2042. http://rsdebate.nic.in/handle/123456789/494625.

'The Mental Health Bill, 1981'. *Rajya Sabha Official Debates, Part 2 – Other than Question and Answer* (25 November 1986): 259–268. http://rsdebate.nic.in/handle/123456789/321321.

The Mental Health Bill, 1981: Report of the Joint Committee. New Delhi: Rajya Sabha Secretariat, 1986.

10. Inside Stories

Ahmed, Farzand, and Avirook Sen. 'Many Inmates Face a Bleak Future as Their Families Abandon Them'. *India Today*, 15 September 1996.

Anon. 'Mental Asylums Sadly Neglected'. *The Times of India* (Bombay), 27 May 1990.

Kalbag, Chaitanya. 'Ranchi Mansik Arogyashala: A Sad Commentary on Mental Asylums in India'. *India Today*, 15 June 1982.

Khandekar, Sreekant. 'Mentally Ill People Flung into Jail for no Fault of Theirs in Madhya Pradesh'. *India Today*, 30 June 1982.

Mishra, Anjana. 'First Person – Hell of a Cure'. *Manushi*, no. 120 (September–October 2000): 12–16.

Nair, Tara S. 'Growth and Structural Transformation of Newspaper Industry in India: an Empirical Investigation'. *Economic & Political Weekly*, vol. 38, no. 39 (27 September 2003): 4182–4189.

Pillai, Sreedhar. 'Young Woman Brutally Raped in Mental Hospital in Kerala'. *India Today*, 15 October 1981.

Qureshi, Shiraj. 'Best Way to Get Rid? Send Them to an Asylum'. *Indian Express* (Madras), 17 June 1994.

Rai, Usha, and Siraj Qureshi. 'Holed in at Agra Mental Hospital – 1: A Dumping Ground for Unwanted Relatives'. *Indian Express* (Madras), 10 July 1994.

Rai, Usha. 'Holed in at Agra Mental Hospital – 2: Sane Millionaire Incarcerated Since 32 Years'. *Indian Express* (Madras), 11 July 1994.

———. 'Holed in at Agra Mental Hospital – 3: Doctors Must Learn the Ethics of Their Profession'. *Indian Express* (Madras), 12 July 1994.

Sengupta, Uttam. 'Asylum Affairs Require Thorough Probe'. *The Telegraph*, 20 September 1984.

———. 'Bodies Pile up at Asylum'. *The Telegraph*, 9 September 1984.

———. 'Mental Asylum a Den of Vice'. *The Telegraph*, 13 September 1984.

_____. 'The Asylum from which the Inmates Escaped'. *The Telegraph*, 8 September 1984.

Vinayak, Ramesh. 'Gross Defect in Law Condemns Inmates of an Amritsar Asylum to Indefinite Detention'. *India Today*, 15 May 1992.

11. Breaking the Law

Akbar, M.J. 'If the Price to be Paid for Publishing these Pictures is a Trip to Jail, So Be It'. *The Telegraph*, 17 February 1983.

_____. 'If You Have Tears, Mr Basu, Shed them for these Inmates of Dum Dum Central Jail …' *The Telegraph*, 17 February 1983.

Anon. 'Who Will Pay for Destroying 54 Yrs of this Man's Life?' *Indian Express* (Bombay), 14 October 2005.

Calcutta High Court. *Rajesh Khaitan vs State of West Bengal and Ors.* Order dated 1 March 1983.

_____. *Rajesh Khaitan vs State of West Bengal and Ors.* Order dated 24 February 1983. https://indiankanoon.org/doc/1455117.

Chadha, Kumkum. *The Indian Jail: A Contemporary Document.* New Delhi: Vikas Publishing House, 1983.

Das, Tapan. 'Dumdum Central Jail: If there is Hell on Earth, it is this, it is this …' *Sunday*, 13 February 1983.

Delhi High Court. *Charanjit Singh and National Human Rights Commission vs State and Ors.* Judgment dated 4 March 2005. https://indiankanoon.org/doc/1230647/.

Ganguly, Tarun. 'Conditions at Dum Dum Central Jail'. *The Telegraph*, 1 February 1983.

Ghosh, Barun, and Umesh Anand. 'Terror Behind Bars'. *The Telegraph*, 16 January 1983.

'Lunatic Asylums'. *Lok Sabha Debates*, vol. LI, no. 13 (3 March 1966): 3571–3572.

Murthy, Srinivasa, and Amita Dhanda. *Unlock the Padlock: Mental Health Care in West Bengal. Report presented to the Supreme Court of India in the matter of Sheela Barse v. Union of India WP (Cri) 237 of 1989.* 1993.

National Crime Records Bureau. *Prison Statistics: 2000*. New Delhi: NCRB, Ministry of Home Affairs, Government of India, 2002.

National Crime Records Bureau. *Prison Statistics India: 2001*. New Delhi: NCRB, Ministry of Home Affairs, Government of India, 2004.

National Human Rights Commission. *National Human Rights Commission: Annual Report 2005–2006*. New Delhi: NHRC, 2006.

Report of National Expert Committee on Women Prisoners. New Delhi: Government of India, Ministry of Human Resource Development, Department of Women and Child Development, 1987.

Report of the All India Committee on Jail Reform 1980–83, Volume 1. Delhi: Ministry of Home Affairs, Government of India, 1983.

Subramanium, Gopal. *Justicia Virtutum Regina. Report of Gopal Subramanium, Senior Advocate, Supreme Court of India. Commissioner appointed by the Hon'ble Supreme Court of India vide order dated 13.5.1994 in Writ petition (Criminal) no 237 of 1989 Sheela Barse vs. Union of India and Another*. 1994.

Supreme Court of India. *Mrs. Veena Sethi vs State Of Bihar and Ors.* Order dated 11 May 1982. https://indiankanoon.org/doc/1928844/.

12. Hope for Hospitals

Kothari, Miloon. 'India's Contribution to the Universal Declaration on Human Rights'. *Journal of the National Human Rights Commission, India*, vol. 17 (2018): 65–98.

Nagaraja, D., and Pratima Murthy, eds. *Mental Health Care and Human Rights*. New Delhi: National Human Rights Commission of India, 2008.

National Human Rights Commission of India. *Quality Assurance in Mental Health*. New Delhi: NHRC, 1999.

Pathare, Soumitra, and Arjun Kapoor. 'Implementation Update on Mental Healthcare Act, 2017'. In *India's Mental Healthcare Act,*

2017: Building Laws, Protecting Rights, by R.M. Duffy and B.D. Kelly, 251–265. Singapore: Springer Nature Singapore Pte Ltd, 2020.

Supreme Court of India. *Mrs. Veena Sethi vs State Of Bihar and Ors.* Order dated 11 May 1982. https://indiankanoon.org/doc/1928844/.

———. *Rakesh Chandra Narayan vs State Of Bihar*. Judgement dated 27 September 1988. https://main.sci.gov.in/jonew/judis/8161.pdf.

———. *Rakesh Chandra Narayan vs State Of Bihar and Ors*. Order dated 8 September 1994. https://indiankanoon.org/doc/1090348/.

'The Mental Healthcare Act, 2017'. *Gazette of India (Extraordinary)*, part II, section 1, no. 10 (7 April 2017).

13. Are We There Yet?

Gururaj G, et al. *National Mental Health Survey of India, 2015–16: Summary*. NIMHANS Publication No. 128. Bengaluru: National Institute of Mental Health and Neuro Sciences, 2016.

Matloff, Judith, and Robert Neckelsberg. 'Beyond the Breaking Point'. Dart Center for Journalism and Trauma, 9 April 2009. https://dartcenter.org/content/beyond-breaking-point.

Tata Trusts. *Pathways of Hope: Stories of Courage; a Journey in Mental Health and Wellness*. Mumbai: Sir Dorabji Tata Trust, 2017.

World Health Organization. *Mental Health Atlas 2017*. Geneva: World Health Organization, 2018. Country profiles available at https://www.who.int/mental_health/evidence/atlas/profiles-2017/en/.

Acknowledgements

In 2017, I submitted a research proposal to the Jawaharlal Nehru Memorial Fund. To my surprise, it earned me a two-year fellowship to write *Asylum*. The expedition had actually begun a couple of years earlier. Now that I was backed by an institution of eminence, I was able to push ahead with greater clarity and purpose.

My search for material started with the annual reports of mental hospitals in colonial India. I found most of them in an unexpected place – the website of the National Library of Scotland. Others were available at the Nehru Memorial Museum & Library. I should mention that while Burma was administered as a province of British India from 1886 to 1937, I came across little information on the mental hospital at Rangoon. So I decided to leave it out. Some annual reports of mental hospitals are terse and dry. But others are detailed, reflective, and beautifully written. Sadly, such reports became extinct in independent India.

The partition of India had left hundreds of Indian patients stranded for years in mental hospitals in Pakistan. Their fate is largely unknown. Relevant reports of the hospitals in question are simply not available – in India, that is. Fortunately, Fakir Aijazuddin sent some of them across from Pakistan. The annual reports of the mental hospital at Lahore from 1947 to 1950 fill in many of the blanks in what we know about the disturbing events of the time.

It was Shilpi Rajpal who convinced me to visit the National Archives of India. The staff taught me how to navigate the massive collection in their care. I spent several weeks poring over delicate archival documents. While it was disappointing when a certain file was either 'missing' or too 'brittle' to be issued, dozens of others made up for that.

Arvind Abraham and Raghav Tankha – my nephew – helped me to find and to decode a variety of legal documents. Gopal Subramanium took a great deal of trouble to unearth a crucial report that he had written at the behest of the Supreme Court. The full story behind the Mental Healthcare Act of 2017 has not yet been told. But I did get some snippets from Keshav Desiraju, then a senior official in the health ministry, and a prime mover of the bill.

The digital media abounds with articles on mental health. Justine Siddiqui put together a large assortment for me. I had to look elsewhere for older articles. Roopinder Singh dug out issues of *The Tribune* from the 1950s. Sakti Roy retrieved the iconic coverage in *The Telegraph* and *Sunday* during the 1980s. And Shripati Ankolekar traced early pieces carried by *The Times of India.* I had the privilege of speaking with Uttam Sengupta, Usha Rai, and Chaitanya Kalbag, whose reportage had made quite a stir in its time. I also spoke with Raghu Rai, whose photographs added volumes to Chaitanya Kalbag's text.

Among all those who helped me, I owe special thanks to Utpal Sarkar at the National Human Rights Commission, Manju Sharma and Kamal Chaurasia at the Lok Sabha Secretariat, and Ramphal Pawar at the National Crime Records Bureau.

Various people have asked me which hospitals I studied at close quarters. The answer is 'none'. I chose to rely on studies conducted by qualified professionals. I did, however, make a trip to Ranchi, which was very kindly arranged by Dr Boniface

Hembrom. As I walked through the picturesque campus, two patients came up and asked me whether I was a patient or a visitor. When I told them that I was a researcher, the two men nodded and strolled off. It was an unexpected start to a rewarding visit. Even before I showed up, the librarian, Jitendra Kumar, had put together a big pile of useful books and reports for me to consult. I had an absorbing conversation with Dr Varun Mehta. And Dr Daya Ram, the director, was more than forthcoming.

Other visits were less rewarding. Muvendran, the librarian at Madras, tried his best to help, but the library had little to offer. He did, however, ply me with numerous cups of tea. My visit came to an end when a suspicious faculty member showed up and virtually shooed me away. Meanwhile, I wrote – twice – to the director's office at Kanke. I did not receive a reply.

My original plan was to meet with a cross-section of people who are engaged in alternative approaches to mental healthcare. I also hoped to reflect the perspective of those who are affected by mental illness. Unfortunately, the Covid-19 pandemic did not allow me to do so.

I could not have written this book without Dr Alok Sarin. He helped me to appreciate the complexity of mental healthcare, and encouraged me to find my own point of view. I am also indebted to Dr Karan Singh, Suman Dubey, and Dr N. Balakrishnan at the Jawaharlal Memorial Fund for their constant support.

Asylum may not have been published without the keen interest taken by Karthika V.K. at Westland. The editing by Sonia Madan, the typesetting by Rajinder Ganju, the index prepared by Gour Sundar Saha, and the cover design by Saurabh Garge and Gavin Morris have given the book the elegance it deserved.

Ashok Patnaik is always the first person to read anything that I write. He is also my husband. I could not have survived this expedition without him.